QUICK AND SIMPLE

Chair Yoga

for seniors over 70:

A Step-by-Step Guide with Gentle Exercise For Elderly Men, Women and Beginners To Reclaim Balance, Improve Mobility and Strength, Transform Their Body And Mind With Adapted Poses.

BY

Dr. Sheila Douglas

BONUS TIP: 21 DAYS CHALLENGE OF YOGA FOR WEIGHT LOSS AND 65 QUICK AND SIMPLE CHAIR EXERCISES TO PERFORM ON THE CHAIR FOR SENIORS BALANCE AND STABILITY.

Table of Contents

Introduction

Welcome to a journey of self-discovery and transformation, where every breath, every movement, and every moment is an invitation to embrace the fullness of your being. In the pages that follow, you'll embark on an adventure into the enriching world of chair yoga, tailored specifically for you – a senior over 70 seeking to unlock the secrets to vitality, wellness, and inner peace.

Imagine yourself seated comfortably in a chair, surrounded by the gentle hum of life's rhythms and the promise of new beginnings. This is where your journey begins – in a space of possibility, where age is not a limitation but a gateway to deeper wisdom and connection.

As you turn the pages of this book, you'll discover the transformative power of chair yoga – a practice that honors your body, mind, and spirit exactly as they are. Through gentle movements, breath awareness, and relaxation techniques, you'll learn how to nurture your physical health, calm your mind, and awaken to the inherent joy and vitality within you.

But this journey is about more than just the poses and practices – it's about embracing a new way of being in the world. It's about cultivating self-compassion, finding gratitude in the simple moments, and fostering a sense of connection to yourself and the world around you.

So, dear reader, are you ready to embark on this journey of self-discovery and transformation? Are you ready to dive deep into the heart of chair yoga and uncover the radiant spirit that lies within? If so, then let us begin. Your adventure awaits, and the possibilities are endless.

Chapter 1:

Introduction to Chair Yoga

Chair yoga is a gentle form of yoga practice that adapts traditional yoga poses and techniques to be performed while seated or with the support of a chair.

It is designed to make yoga accessible to individuals with limited mobility, balance concerns, or physical disabilities, making it suitable for seniors, office workers, individual's recovering from injuries, and anyone else who may benefit from a more gentle approach to yoga.

Chair yoga typically includes modified poses, gentle stretches, breath awareness exercises, and relaxation techniques, all of which can help improve flexibility, strength, posture, and overall well-being.

Welcome, dear reader, to your journey into the enriching world of chair yoga. As a senior over 70, you're embarking on a path of self-discovery, wellness, and vitality.

In this chapter, we'll lay the groundwork for your chair yoga practice, exploring its benefits and guiding you through the first steps of your transformative journey.

Imagine yourself sitting comfortably in a chair, feet planted firmly on the ground, spine tall and straight. This is where your journey begins – in a place of stability and support. Chair yoga is a gentle form of yoga specially designed for individuals with limited mobility, making it perfect for seniors like yourself.

As you take a moment to settle into your seat, let's delve into the essence of chair yoga. Unlike traditional yoga practices that require you to perform poses on a mat, chair yoga allows you to experience the benefits of yoga while seated or using the chair for support. This accessibility makes it ideal for seniors who may face challenges with balance, flexibility, or mobility.

Now, close your eyes and take a deep breath-in, filling your lungs with fresh, revitalizing air. With each exhale, release any tension or worries you may be holding onto. In chair yoga, the breath is your constant companion, guiding you through each movement and anchoring you in the present moment.

One of the greatest gifts of chair yoga is its ability to promote physical, mental, and emotional well-being.

Through gentle stretches, mindful breathing, and relaxation techniques, you'll discover a renewed sense of vitality and peace. From improving flexibility and strength to reducing stress and anxiety, the benefits of chair yoga are truly transformative.

But perhaps the most beautiful aspect of chair yoga is its inclusivity. Regardless of your age, fitness level, or physical condition, chair yoga welcomes you with open arms. Whether you're recovering from an injury, managing a chronic health condition, or simply seeking a gentle way to stay active, chair yoga offers something for everyone.

As you begin your chair yoga practice, remember to approach it with an open heart and a curious mind. Embrace each moment as an opportunity to nurture your body, calm your mind, and connect with your inner self. With dedication and patience, you'll gradually unfold the layers of your practice, revealing the radiant spirit that lies within.

1.1 How to Begin a Chair Yoga Practice

Embarking on a journey into chair yoga for seniors is a gentle yet profound step towards enhancing your physical and mental well-being. As you start, find a comfortable chair that supports your back and allows your feet to rest flat on the floor. Sit with your spine tall and your shoulders relaxed.

Begin your practice with a few moments of mindful breathing, focusing on inhaling deeply through your nose and exhaling slowly through your mouth. This sets the tone for a calm and centered practice.

Next, engage in gentle warm-up movements to awaken your body and prepare it for the yoga postures to come. You might start with neck rolls, gently rotating your head in circles to release tension. Then, move on to shoulder shrugs, rolling your shoulders forward and backward to loosen any stiffness.

These simple movements help improve circulation and flexibility, priming your body for the practice ahead.

1.2 How Is Chair Yoga Performed?

Chair yoga offers a gentle yet effective way to experience the benefits of traditional yoga poses while seated or using the chair for support. As you engage in chair yoga, focus on your breath and move mindfully, allowing your breath to guide your movements. Explore a range of seated poses, such as seated twists, forward folds, and gentle backbends, adapting them to your comfort level and physical abilities.

Throughout your practice, maintain awareness of your alignment, ensuring that your spine remains elongated and your joints are in a safe and stable position. Use the chair for support as needed, whether by resting your hands on the seat for balance or using it as a prop for deeper stretches.

1.3 Who Can Practice Chair Yoga?

Chair yoga is accessible to individuals of all ages and fitness levels, making it an ideal practice for seniors. Whether you're new to yoga or have been practicing for years, chair yoga offers a gentle yet effective way to improve flexibility, strength, and overall well-being. It's particularly beneficial for seniors who may have mobility issues or difficulty getting down on the floor for traditional yoga poses.

If you're recovering from an injury or managing a chronic condition, chair yoga can provide a safe and supportive way to stay active and maintain your health. Additionally, chair yoga offers mental benefits, such as stress reduction and improved focus, making it a valuable practice for seniors looking to enhance their quality of life.

1.4 Health Benefits for Seniors Performing Yoga

The health benefits of chair yoga for seniors are vast and varied, encompassing physical, mental, and emotional well-being. Regular practice can help improve flexibility, range of motion, and balance, reducing the risk of falls and enhancing overall mobility.

Chair yoga also strengthens muscles and bones, supporting healthy aging and reducing the risk of osteoporosis.

Beyond the physical benefits, chair yoga offers mental and emotional support for seniors. It promotes relaxation and stress reduction, helping to alleviate anxiety and depression.

By focusing on the present moment and cultivating mindfulness, chair yoga fosters a sense of inner peace and contentment, enhancing overall quality of life.

Getting started with chair yoga for seniors is a journey of self-discovery and self-care. By following these steps and embracing the practice with an open heart and mind, you can experience the transformative power of yoga in your life. So, take a seat, breathe deeply, and let the healing journey begin.

1.5 Watch Out For Safety Measures

Before we launch into the depth of this gems, safety is paramount in any yoga practice, especially for seniors. Before beginning chair yoga, it's essential to consult with your healthcare provider, especially if you have any existing medical conditions or physical limitations. Once you have the green light to proceed, listen to your body throughout your practice and honor its signals. Avoid pushing yourself into discomfort or pain, and modify poses as needed to suit your individual needs.

When practicing chair yoga, ensure that your chair is stable and secure, with no wobbling or risk of tipping over. Place your chair on a flat surface, away from any obstacles that could interfere with your movements. Additionally, use props such as yoga blocks or cushions to provide support and make poses more accessible.

Watch Tutorial videos: Click here https://youtu.be/4-wpPBQZ-as?si=A8bZ9XgJ3XPoD5c6

Chapter 2:

Setting the Foundation

Now that you've been introduced to the concept of chair yoga, it's time to lay the foundation for your practice.

Find a quiet, comfortable space where you can dedicate time to yourself without distractions. Settle into your chair, adjusting your posture so that your feet are firmly planted on the ground and your spine is tall and straight.

Before we delve into the physical aspects of chair yoga, let's take a moment to center ourselves through the breath. Close your eyes and bring your awareness to your breath, feeling the gentle rise and fall of your chest with each inhale and exhale.

Allow your breath to become slow, deep, and steady, grounding you in the present moment.

As you continue to breathe mindfully, take a moment to set an intention for your practice. What do you hope to achieve through chair yoga? Whether it's increasing flexibility, reducing stress, or simply finding moments of peace amidst the busyness of life, let your intention guide you as you move through your practice.

Now, let's explore the importance of proper alignment in chair yoga. Situate yourself towards the front edge of your chair, allowing your hips to be slightly higher than your knees.

WATCH TUTORIAL VIDEOS:
https://youtu.be/U_jdXFfegKE?si=9m2sXqlSzLaqHdA3

This alignment helps to maintain the natural curve of your spine and prevents slouching. Roll your shoulders back and down, opening up the chest and allowing for easier breathing.

As you settle into this aligned position, take a moment to scan your body for any areas of tension or discomfort. If you notice any tightness or pain, gently adjust your posture or use props such as cushions or blankets for added support.

Remember, your comfort and safety are paramount in your yoga practice.

With your foundation set and your body aligned, you're now ready to begin your journey into the heart of chair yoga.

The Major Styles of Chair Yoga

2.1 The Integral Yoga

Integral yoga is a holistic approach to yoga that incorporates asanas (poses), pranayama (breath-work), meditation, and self-inquiry to promote health and well-being. Rooted in the teachings of Sri Swami Satchidananda, integral yoga aims to integrate the body, mind, and spirit, fostering a sense of wholeness and unity.

As you engage in integral chair yoga, focus on cultivating awareness and presence, embracing each moment with openness and acceptance.

Integral chair yoga offers a diverse range of practices, from gentle stretching and relaxation to more dynamic sequences and meditation techniques. Explore the various aspects of integral yoga, discovering which practices resonate most deeply with you.

Whether you're seeking physical fitness, stress relief, or spiritual growth, integral chair yoga offers a comprehensive approach to wellness for seniors.

2.2 The Core-Power Yoga

Core-Power yoga is a modern style of yoga that combines dynamic movement, strength-building exercises, and breath-work to create a challenging and invigorating practice. With a focus on building core strength and endurance, Core-Power yoga offers a full-body workout that leaves you feeling energized and empowered. As you engage in Core-Power chair yoga, focus on connecting with your breath and engaging your core muscles with each movement.

The Core-Power chair yoga incorporates a variety of poses and sequences, from flowing vinyasa sequences to intense core-focused exercises.

Explore the dynamic interplay between strength and flexibility, pushing your limits while honoring your body's needs. Core-Power chair yoga is a great way for seniors to build strength, improve balance, and boost overall fitness levels, supporting healthy aging and vitality.

2.3 The Power Yoga

Power yoga is a vigorous and dynamic style of yoga that emphasizes strength, flexibility, and endurance. With a focus on flowing sequences and challenging poses, power yoga offers a high-intensity workout that builds heat and sweat. As you engage in power chair yoga, focus on connecting with your breath and staying present in each moment, embracing the physical and mental challenge of the practice.

Power chair yoga offers a diverse range of poses and sequences, from intense sun salutations to challenging arm balances and inversions. Explore the balance between effort and ease, pushing your limits while maintaining awareness of your body's signals. Power chair yoga is a great way for seniors to build strength, increase flexibility, and cultivate mental resilience, supporting overall health and well-being.

2.4 Hatha Yoga

The Hatha yoga is a traditional style of yoga that focuses on the balance between body and mind through physical postures (asanas) and breath control (pranayama).

With a gentle approach to movement and an emphasis on alignment and breath awareness, Hatha yoga is accessible to practitioners of all levels, including seniors. As you engage in Hatha chair yoga, focus on cultivating a sense of ease and stability in each pose, finding the balance between effort and relaxation.

Hatha chair yoga offers a variety of poses and sequences, from gentle stretches to more challenging balances and twists. Explore the full range of motion in your body, moving with awareness and intention. Pay attention to your breath, using it as a guide to deepen into poses and release tension. Hatha chair yoga is a great way for seniors to improve flexibility, balance, and overall well-being, promoting a sense of harmony and vitality.

2.5 The Restorative Yoga

Restorative yoga is a gentle and nurturing style of yoga that focuses on relaxation and rejuvenation. With an emphasis on supported poses and deep relaxation techniques, restorative yoga helps calm the nervous system, reduce stress, and promote healing.

As you engage in restorative chair yoga, focus on surrendering to the support of props such as blankets, bolsters, and blocks, allowing your body to release tension and unwind.

The Restorative chair yoga offers a series of passive poses held for extended periods, allowing you to fully relax and let go. Explore the sensation of being fully supported and held, sinking deeper into a state of relaxation with each breath. Restorative chair yoga is a wonderful way for seniors to soothe sore muscles, calm the mind, and restore balance to the body, promoting deep relaxation and rejuvenation.

2.6 The Half Sun Salutation

The half sun salutation is a simplified version of the traditional sun salutation sequence, making it accessible to seniors and beginners. With a focus on gentle movement and breath awareness, the half sun salutation helps warm up the body and awaken energy.

As you engage in the half sun salutation in a chair, focus on connecting with your breath and moving with ease and fluidity.

Begin in a seated position with your feet flat on the floor and your spine tall. Inhale, reaching your arms overhead, and exhale, folding forward with a straight back. Inhale, lifting your torso halfway up, and exhale, folding forward again.

Inhale, sweeping your arms out to the sides and up overhead, and exhale, bringing your hands back to your heart center. Repeat the sequence several times, moving with your breath and enjoying the gentle flow of movement.

2.7 Prenatal Yoga

Prenatal yoga is a specialized form of chair yoga designed to support pregnant women during all stages of pregnancy.

With a focus on gentle movements, breath awareness, and relaxation techniques, prenatal yoga helps expectant mothers stay active, relieve discomfort, and prepare for childbirth. As you engage in prenatal chair yoga, focus on connecting with your baby and nurturing your body, mind, and spirit.

Throughout your practice, listen to your body and honor its needs, modifying poses as needed to accommodate your changing body. Focus on deep, mindful breathing to reduce stress and promote relaxation, easing tension and anxiety. Prenatal chair yoga can also help alleviate common pregnancy symptoms such as back pain, swelling, and fatigue, leaving you feeling refreshed and rejuvenated.

2.8 The Optimal Relaxation Chair Yoga Routine for seniors

An optimal relaxation chair yoga routine for seniors offers a series of gentle stretches, breath-work, and relaxation techniques to promote deep relaxation and stress relief.

Begin by finding a comfortable seated position in your chair, with your feet flat on the floor and your spine tall. Close your eyes and take a few deep breaths, allowing your body and mind to settle into the present moment.

Start with gentle neck stretches, tilting your head from side to side and gently rolling it in circles to release tension. Then, move on to shoulder rolls, lifting your shoulders up towards your ears and then rolling them back and down.

Continue with gentle twists and side stretches, moving with your breath and exploring the full range of motion in your body.

After warming up your body, transition into deep relaxation poses such as supported forward folds and reclining twists. Use props such as blankets and bolsters to support your body and promote comfort.

Focus on releasing tension with each exhalation, sinking deeper into relaxation with each breath.

Finish your relaxation routine with a few minutes of guided meditation or deep breathing exercises.

Allow yourself to fully let go and surrender to the present moment, experiencing a profound sense of peace and tranquility. As you emerge from your practice, take a moment to notice how your body and mind feel, appreciating the profound benefits of relaxation chair yoga for seniors.

2.9 The Best Yoga Poses for Bedtime To Help You Sleep Better

Yoga poses can be incredibly beneficial for promoting relaxation and preparing the body for sleep. Incorporating gentle yoga poses into your bedtime routine can help calm the nervous system, reduce stress, and promote a sense of ease and relaxation.

Here are some of the best yoga poses for bedtime to help you sleep better:

- **Legs-Up-the-Wall Pose (Viparita Karani):** This restorative pose helps calm the mind, relieve tension in the legs, and promote relaxation.

Lie on your back with your legs extended up against a wall, forming a gentle inversion. Close your eyes and focus on your breath as you relax into the pose for several minutes.

- **Child's Pose (Balasana):** This gentle forward fold helps release tension in the back, shoulders, and hips, promoting relaxation and stress relief.

Begin on your hands and knees, then sit back on your heels and fold forward, resting your forehead on the floor and extending your arms out in front of you. Breathe deeply and surrender to the pose for several breaths.

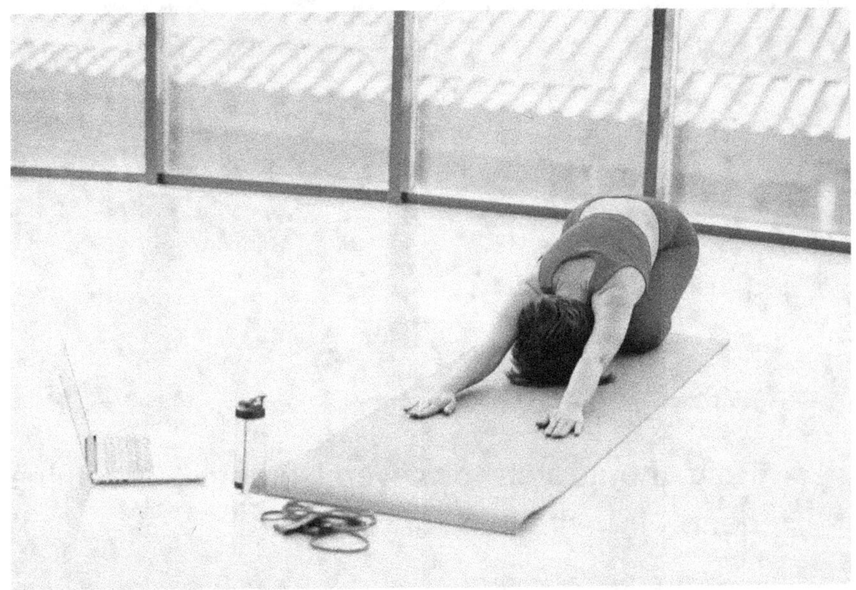

- **Seated Forward Bend** (Paschimottanasana): This seated stretch helps calm the mind, release tension in the back and hamstrings, and promote relaxation. Sit on the edge of a chair with your legs extended in front of you, then hinge forward at the hips and reach towards your feet, allowing your spine to lengthen and your head to drop towards your knees.

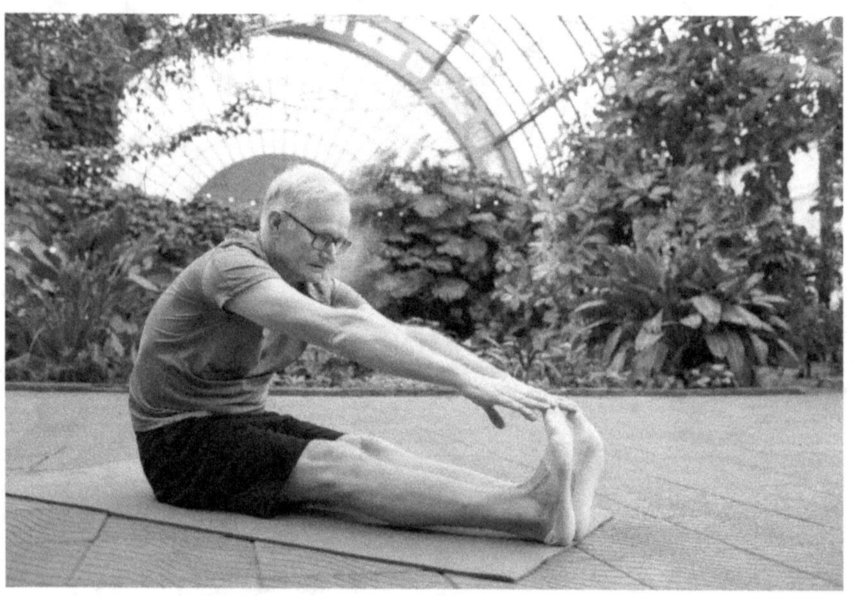

- Hold the stretch for several breaths, breathing deeply into the back of your body.

- **Reclining Bound Angle Pose (Supta Baddha Konasana):** This restorative pose helps open the hips and chest, promote relaxation, and prepare the body for sleep. Lie on your back with the soles of your feet together and your knees falling open to the sides, forming a diamond shape with your legs. Place a bolster or folded blanket under your spine for support, allowing your arms to rest at your sides with your palms facing up. Close your eyes and breathe deeply into your belly, surrendering to the pose for several minutes.

- **Corpse Pose (Savasana)**: This final relaxation pose helps calm the mind, release tension throughout the body, and promote deep relaxation.

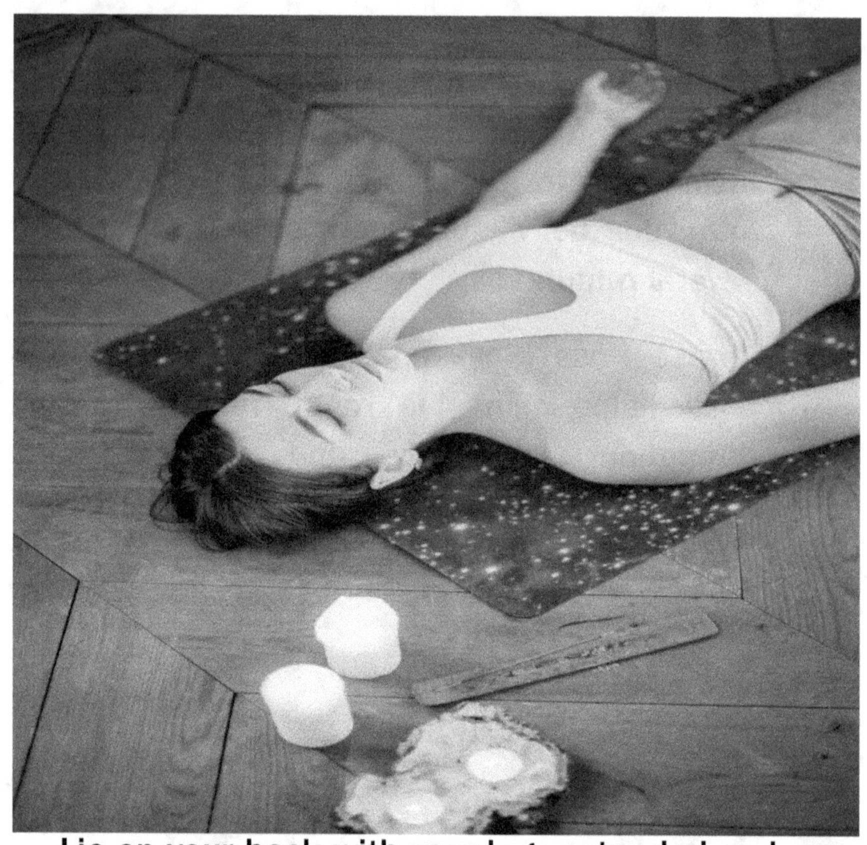

Lie on your back with your legs extended and your arms resting at your sides, palms facing up. Close your eyes and allow your body to relax completely, surrendering to the support of the earth beneath you. Focus on your breath as you let go of any tension or stress, allowing yourself to sink into a state of deep relaxation.

Incorporating these gentle yoga poses into your bedtime routine can help calm your mind, release tension from your body, and prepare you for a restful night's sleep.

Practice them regularly to experience the profound benefits of yoga for sleep and overall well-being.

➤ *Bedtime Wind-Down Tips*

In addition to practicing gentle yoga poses before bed, there are several other bedtime wind-down tips that can help promote relaxation and prepare your body and mind for sleep.

Here are some suggestions to incorporate into your nightly routine:

Create a soothing bedtime ritual: Establishing a calming bedtime routine can signal to your body that it's time to wind down and prepare for sleep. This could include activities such as taking a warm bath, practicing gentle yoga or meditation, reading a book, or listening to calming music.

Limit screen time: Excessive exposure to screens, such as smartphones, tablets, and computers, can interfere with your body's natural sleep-wake cycle and make it harder to fall asleep. Aim to power down electronic devices at least an hour before bed to give your brain time to unwind and transition into sleep mode.

Create a comfortable sleep environment: Make sure your bedroom is conducive to sleep by keeping it cool, dark, and quiet. Invest in a comfortable mattress and pillows that support your body and promote proper alignment. Consider using blackout curtains or a white noise machine to block out any distractions that could disrupt your sleep.

Practice relaxation techniques: Incorporate relaxation techniques such as deep breathing, progressive muscle relaxation, or guided imagery into your bedtime routine to help calm your mind and relax your body.

These techniques can help reduce stress and tension, making it easier to fall asleep and stay asleep throughout the night.

Limit caffeine and alcohol: Avoid consuming caffeine and alcohol in the hours leading up to bedtime, as they can interfere with your ability to fall asleep and stay asleep. Instead, opt for herbal teas or warm milk, which can promote relaxation and help prepare your body for sleep.

Practice gratitude: Take a few moments before bed to reflect on the positive aspects of your day and express gratitude for the blessings in your life. Cultivating a sense of gratitude can help shift your focus away from worries and stressors, promoting a sense of peace and contentment that can aid in falling asleep more easily.

By incorporating these bedtime wind-down tips into your nightly routine, you can create a peaceful and relaxing environment that supports restful sleep. Experiment with different techniques to find what works best for you, and commit to prioritizing your sleep and overall well-being.

2.10 Concerns Regarding Health

While chair yoga can offer numerous benefits for seniors, it's essential to be aware of potential health concerns and take appropriate precautions to ensure a safe and enjoyable practice.

Here are some common concerns regarding health in chair yoga for seniors:

Joint pain and stiffness: Many seniors experience joint pain and stiffness due to arthritis, osteoporosis, or other age-related conditions. It's essential to practice chair yoga mindfully, avoiding movements that exacerbate joint pain and modifying poses as needed to accommodate any limitations. Gentle stretching and range-of-motion exercises can help alleviate stiffness and improve joint mobility over time.

Balance issues: Balance can decline with age, increasing the risk of falls and injuries. When practicing chair yoga, be mindful of your balance and use the chair for support as needed.

Focus on poses that improve balance, such as standing poses with the support of the chair or seated poses that engage the core muscles. Gradually challenge your balance in a safe and controlled manner, but always prioritize safety and stability.

Cardiovascular health: Seniors with cardiovascular issues should approach chair yoga with caution, especially if they have high blood pressure or heart disease.

Avoid rapid or strenuous movements that could elevate heart rate or blood pressure to unsafe levels. Instead, focus on gentle, controlled movements and incorporate deep breathing exercises to promote relaxation and stress reduction.

Breathing difficulties: Seniors with respiratory conditions such as asthma or COPD may find certain breathing exercises challenging. It's essential to approach pranayama (breathwork) with caution, starting slowly and gradually increasing intensity as tolerated.

Focus on gentle breathing exercises that promote relaxation and improve lung function, such as diaphragmatic breathing or alternate nostril breathing.

Injuries: Seniors may be more prone to injuries due to age-related changes in musculoskeletal health and mobility. It's crucial to practice chair yoga mindfully, paying attention to alignment and avoiding overexertion or pushing beyond your limits. Listen to your body and honor its signals, modifying poses as needed to prevent strain or injury.

By being mindful of these potential health concerns and taking appropriate precautions, seniors can enjoy the numerous benefits of chair yoga while minimizing the risk of injury or discomfort. Remember to consult with your healthcare provider before beginning any new exercise program, especially if you have any pre-existing health conditions or concerns.

2.11 Options for Beginners

For seniors who are new to chair yoga, it's essential to start slowly and gradually build up strength, flexibility, and confidence in their practice. **Here are some options for beginners to ease into chair yoga:**

- **Gentle stretching:** Begin with simple, gentle stretching exercises to warm up the body and release tension. Focus on areas of the body that feel tight or tense, such as the neck, shoulders, and hips. Move slowly and mindfully, breathing deeply into each stretch and avoiding any pain or discomfort.

- *Seated poses*: Explore a variety of seated yoga poses that can be done comfortably in a chair. Start with basic poses such as seated mountain pose, seated forward fold, and seated twist. Use the chair for support as needed, and focus on alignment and breath awareness in each pose.

- *Breath-work*: Incorporate simple breathing exercises into your practice to promote relaxation and reduce stress. Try diaphragmatic breathing, in which you breathe deeply into your belly, expanding and contracting with each breath. Practice mindful breathing, focusing on the sensation of the breath as it enters and leaves your body.

- ***Meditation:*** Begin or end your practice with a short meditation to calm the mind and cultivate inner peace. Start with just a few minutes of meditation, focusing on your breath or repeating a calming mantra or affirmation. Gradually increase the duration of your meditation as you become more comfortable with the practice.

- ***Chair yoga classes***: Consider joining a chair yoga class specifically designed for seniors or beginners.

A qualified instructor can guide you through gentle sequences and provide modifications and adjustments to suit your individual needs. Plus, practicing in a group setting can provide support, motivation, and a sense of community.

By starting slowly and exploring these beginner-friendly options, seniors can begin their chair yoga journey with confidence and ease. Remember to listen to your body, honor its limits, and enjoy the process of discovering the transformative power of yoga.

When beginning a chair yoga practice, it's essential to start with gentle and safe exercises that gradually introduce movement and stretch to the body.

These starting exercises are designed to be accessible to individuals of all ages and fitness levels, providing a foundation for building strength, flexibility, and mindfulness. Here are some friendly and safe starting exercises to try:

➢ **Seated Cat-Cow Pose:** Sit towards the front of your chair with your feet flat on the floor and your hands resting on your knees. Inhale as you arch your back and lift your chest forward, opening your heart towards the ceiling (Cow Pose). Exhale as you round your spine and tuck your chin towards your chest, drawing your navel towards your spine (Cat Pose). Repeat this flowing movement several times, moving with your breath.

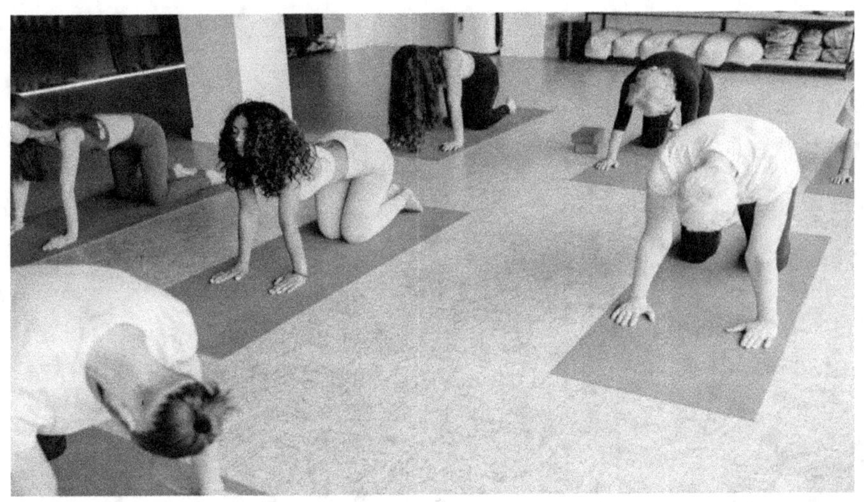

➢ **_Cross-Legged Poses and Their Benefits_**: Sit towards the front of your chair with your feet flat on the floor and your spine tall. Cross your right ankle over your left knee, flexing your right foot to protect your knee. Keep your spine tall and gently press your right knee towards the floor, feeling a stretch through your right hip and outer thigh. Hold for several breaths, then switch sides.

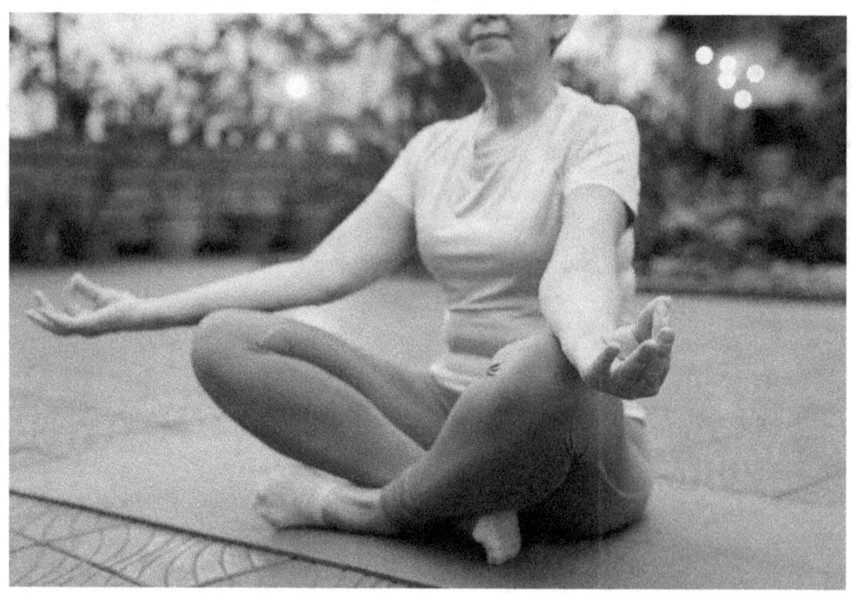

> ***Seated Side Bend Pose Fundamentals:*** Sit tall in your chair with your feet flat on the floor and your hands resting on your thighs. Inhale to lengthen your spine, then exhale to lean to the right, bringing your right hand down towards the floor and reaching your left arm up and over your head. Feel a stretch along the left side of your body. Hold for several breaths, then switch sides.

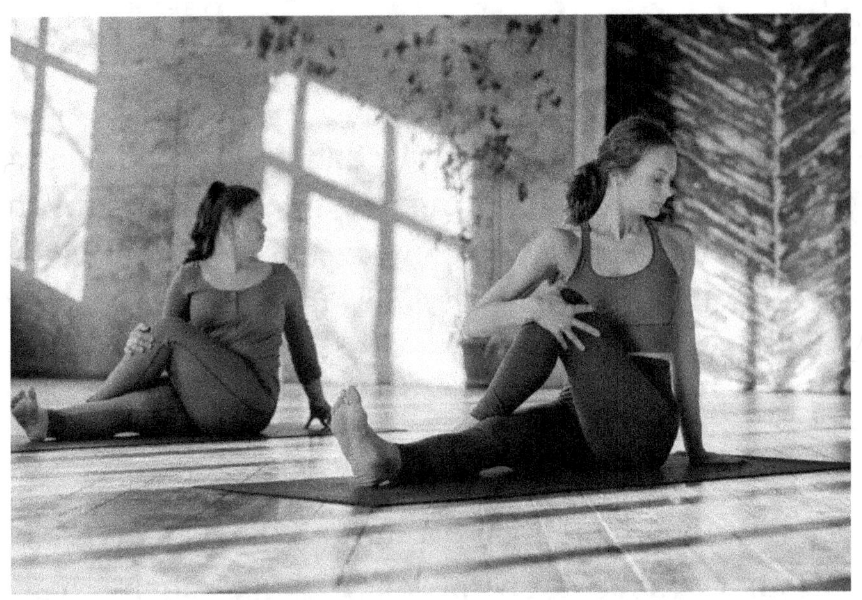

- > ***Ragdoll Pose***: Sit towards the front of your chair with your feet flat on the floor and your spine tall. Inhale to lengthen your spine, then exhale to hinge forward from your hips, bringing your chest towards your thighs. Allow your arms to hang down towards the floor, relaxing your head and neck. Feel a gentle stretch through your spine, hamstrings, and shoulders. Hold for several breaths, then slowly roll back up to a seated position.

By incorporating these friendly and safe starting exercises into your chair yoga practice, you can gradually build strength, flexibility, and mindfulness while reducing tension and stress in the body.

Remember to move mindfully and gently, listening to your body's cues and respecting its limits. With regular practice, you can experience the many benefits of chair yoga and cultivate a greater sense of well-being.

2.13 Cross-Legged Poses and Their Benefits

Cross-legged poses are a staple in yoga practice and offer a range of benefits for the body and mind. Whether practiced on the floor or in a chair, cross-legged poses help to open the hips, stretch the inner thighs, and promote relaxation and mindfulness.

WATCH 15-MINUTE SAMPLE WORKOUT VIDEO :

https://youtu.be/Ev6yE55kYGw?si=oE2ikCQ4OLNwk 5G5

Here are some cross-legged poses and their benefits:

- ➢ **Easy Pose (Sukhasana**): Sit comfortably on the floor or in a chair with your legs crossed and your spine tall. Place your hands on your knees or thighs, palms facing down or up. Close your eyes and take several deep breaths, grounding down through your sit bones and lengthening up through the crown of your head. Easy Pose helps to improve posture, increase hip flexibility, and promote relaxation and calm.

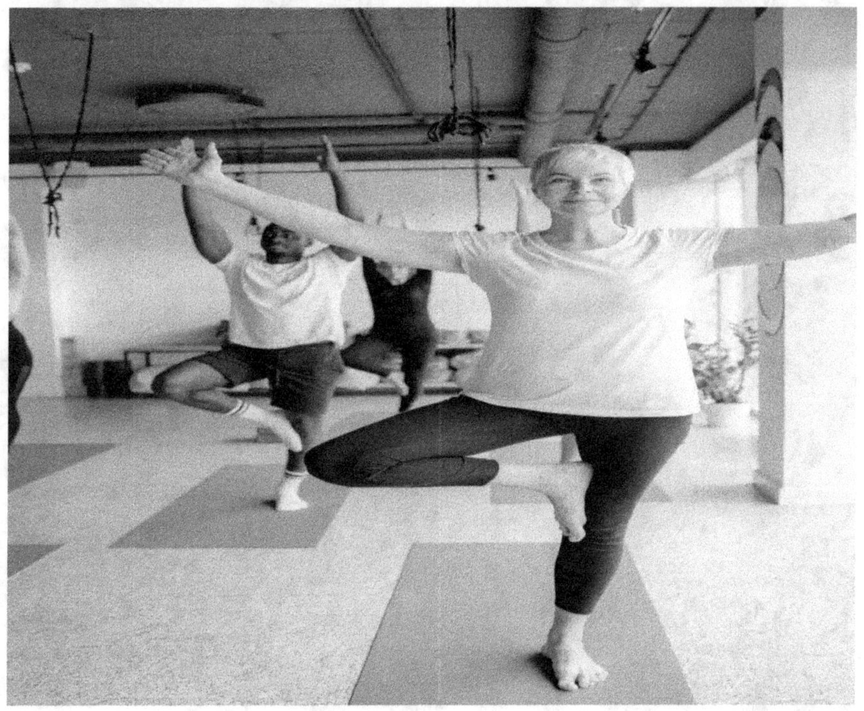

➢ **Half Lotus Pose (Ardha Padmasana):** Sit comfortably on the floor or in a chair with your legs crossed. Bring your right foot towards your left hip crease, allowing your right knee to drop towards the floor.

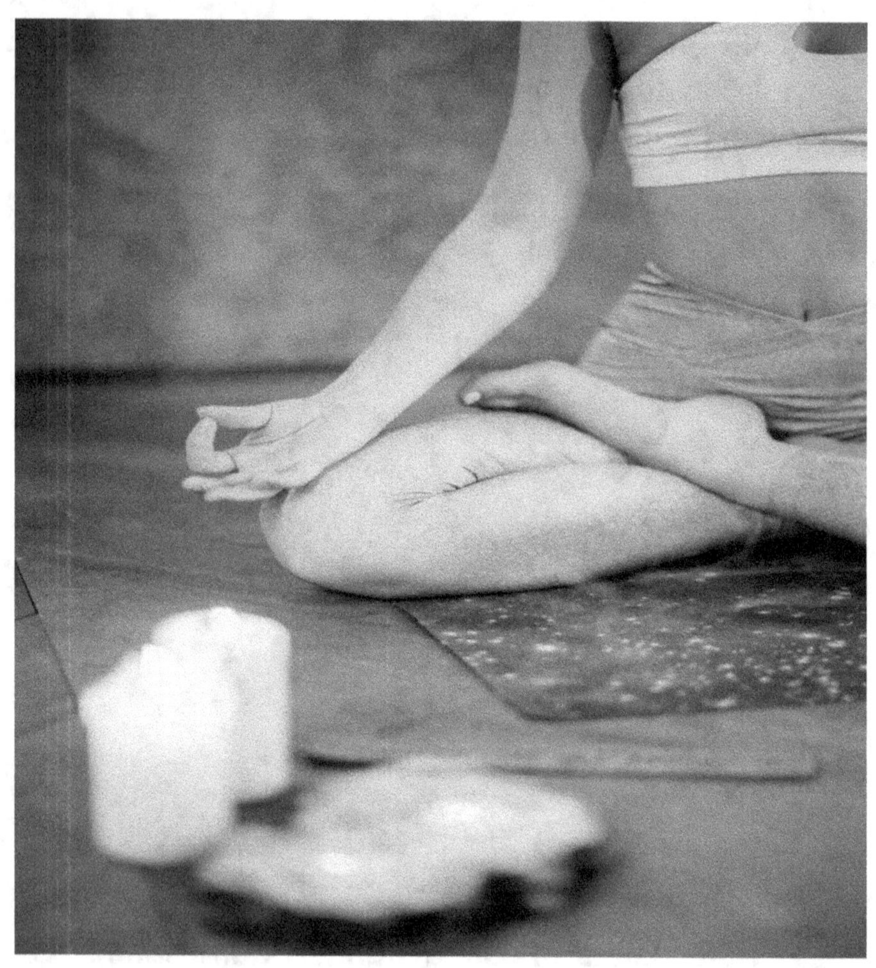

> Keep your left foot on the floor or bring it to rest on top of your right thigh, ankle resting near your hip crease. Place your hands on your knees or thighs and sit tall. Half Lotus Pose helps to stretch the hips, knees, and ankles, and promotes a sense of groundedness and stability.

Full Lotus Pose (Padmasana): Sit comfortably on the floor or in a chair with your legs crossed. Bring both feet towards the opposite hip creases, allowing the knees to drop towards the floor.

Place your hands on your knees or thighs and sit tall. Full Lotus Pose is a more advanced variation of Half Lotus Pose and offers similar benefits, including hip opening, flexibility, and stability.

Seated Cross-Legged Pose: Sit comfortably on the floor or in a chair with your legs crossed and your spine tall. Place your hands on your knees or thighs and sit tall. This simple cross-legged pose helps to open the hips, stretch the inner thighs, and promote relaxation and mindfulness.

It is accessible to individuals of all ages and abilities and can be modified as needed for comfort and support.

2.14 The Seated Side Bend Pose Fundamentals

Seated side bend pose is a gentle yoga pose that stretches the sides of the body, improves spinal mobility, and promotes relaxation and mindfulness. When practiced in a chair, seated side bend pose is accessible to individuals of all ages and abilities, making it an excellent option for beginners and those with limited mobility.

Here's how to practice seated side bend pose:

➤ Sit comfortably in your chair with your feet flat on the floor and your spine tall.

➤ Inhale to lengthen your spine, reaching the crown of your head towards the ceiling.

➤ Exhale to gently lean to the right, bringing your right hand down towards the floor and reaching your left arm up and over your head.

➤ Keep both sit bones grounded on the chair seat and avoid collapsing into the side bend. Instead, imagine lengthening the left side of your body as you reach your left arm towards the right side of the room.

> Hold the stretch for several breaths, feeling a gentle stretch along the left side of your body from your hip to your fingertips.

> Inhale to come back to the center, lengthening your spine once again.

> Exhale as you gently lean to the left, bringing your left hand down towards the floor and reaching your right arm up and over your head.

> Maintain awareness of both sit bones grounding into the chair seat and avoid collapsing into the side bend. Lengthen the right side of your body as you reach your right arm towards the left side of the room.

> Hold the stretch for several breaths, feeling a gentle stretch along the right side of your body from your hip to your fingertips.

➢ Inhale to come back to the center, returning to a neutral seated position.

➢ Repeat the seated side bend pose on each side several times, moving with your breath and maintaining awareness of the sensations in your body.

➢ Seated side bend pose helps to increase flexibility in the spine and side body, improve posture, and relieve tension in the shoulders and neck. It also promotes relaxation and mindfulness by encouraging focused breathing and body awareness.

2.14 The Ragdoll Pose

Ragdoll pose, also known as Uttanasana in traditional yoga, is a relaxing and rejuvenating forward fold that helps to release tension in the spine, hamstrings, and shoulders. When practiced in a chair, ragdoll pose becomes accessible to individuals of all ages and abilities, making it an excellent option for beginners and those with limited mobility.

Here's how to practice ragdoll pose in a chair:

WATCH VIDEO TUTORIAL:

https://youtu.be/G8BsLIPE1m4?si=6LUddIK6IRZYm
U3L

> Sit comfortably towards the front of your chair with your feet flat on the floor and your spine tall.

> Inhale to lengthen your spine, reaching the crown of your head towards the ceiling.

> Exhale as you hinge forward from your hips, bringing your chest towards your thighs and allowing your arms to hang down towards the floor.

> Let your head and neck relax, allowing your chin to tuck towards your chest.

> Allow your spine to round naturally as you deepen into the forward fold, feeling a gentle stretch along the length of your spine.

➢ You can hold onto the legs of the chair, let your hands hang freely, or even clasp opposite elbows with your hands.

➢ Hold the pose for several breaths, allowing gravity to gently pull you deeper into the stretch with each exhale.

➢ To come out of the pose, inhale as you slowly roll back up to a seated position, stacking each vertebra on top of the next.

Ragdoll pose helps to release tension in the spine, shoulders, and neck, improve flexibility in the hamstrings and lower back, and promote relaxation and stress relief. It also encourages mindful breathing and body awareness, making it an excellent addition to any chair yoga practice.

Chapter 3:

Awakening Your Body

As you continue your journey into chair yoga, it's time to awaken your body with gentle movements and stretches. These exercises will help increase circulation, release tension, and prepare your body for the deeper aspects of your practice.

- ➢ Begin by sitting tall in your chair, feet flat on the ground, and hands resting comfortably on your thighs.

- ➢ Take a deep breath in, lengthening your spine, and as you exhale, gently tilt your head to the right, bringing your right ear towards your right shoulder.

- ➢ Feel the stretch along the left side of your neck and hold for a few breaths. Then, return to center and repeat on the opposite side.

- ➢ Next, bring your hands to your shoulders, elbows pointing out to the sides. Inhale as you reach your elbows up towards the ceiling, opening up through the chest.

- ➢ Exhale as you draw your elbows together in front of you, rounding through the upper back.

- ➢ Repeat this movement several times, coordinating your breath with the movement of your arms.

Now, place your hands on the sides of your chair and gently twist your torso to the right, looking over your right shoulder. Keep your hips rooted and your spine tall as you deepen into the twist. Take a few breaths here, feeling the gentle stretch through your spine. Then, return to center and repeat on the left side.

Continue to explore gentle movements and stretches, listening to your body and moving with awareness and ease. Remember to breathe deeply and stay connected to the present moment as you awaken each part of your body.

Advanced Chair Yoga Poses for seniors

3.1 Advanced Chair Yoga Poses for seniors

As you progress in your chair yoga practice, you may feel ready to explore more challenging poses that build strength, flexibility, and balance. Advanced chair yoga poses for seniors offer an opportunity to deepen your practice and continue to reap the benefits of yoga as you age.

Here are some advanced chair yoga poses to try:

- ➤ **Eagle Arms:** Sit tall in your chair and reach your arms out to the sides at shoulder height. Cross your right arm over your left, bringing the backs of your hands together or wrapping your arms around each other until your palms touch.

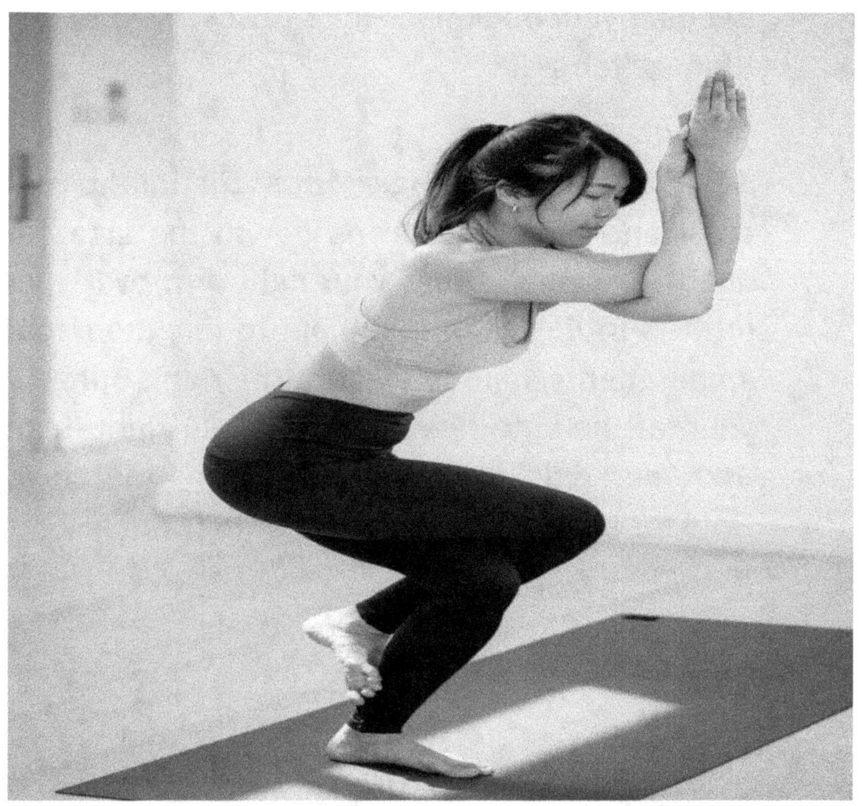

Lift your elbows slightly and feel a stretch across your upper back and shoulders. Hold for several breaths, then switch sides.

> **Chair Pigeon Pose:** Sit towards the front of your chair with your feet flat on the floor. Cross your right ankle over your left knee, flexing your right foot to protect your knee. Keep your spine tall and gently hinge forward from your hips, keeping your back flat. Hold for several breaths, then switch sides.

> **Seated Twist with Eagle Arms:** Sit tall in your chair and bring your arms out to the sides at shoulder height. Cross your right arm over your left, as in Eagle Arms. Inhale to lengthen your spine, then exhale to twist to the right, bringing your left hand to the outside of your right thigh and your right hand to the back of the chair. Hold for several breaths, then switch sides.

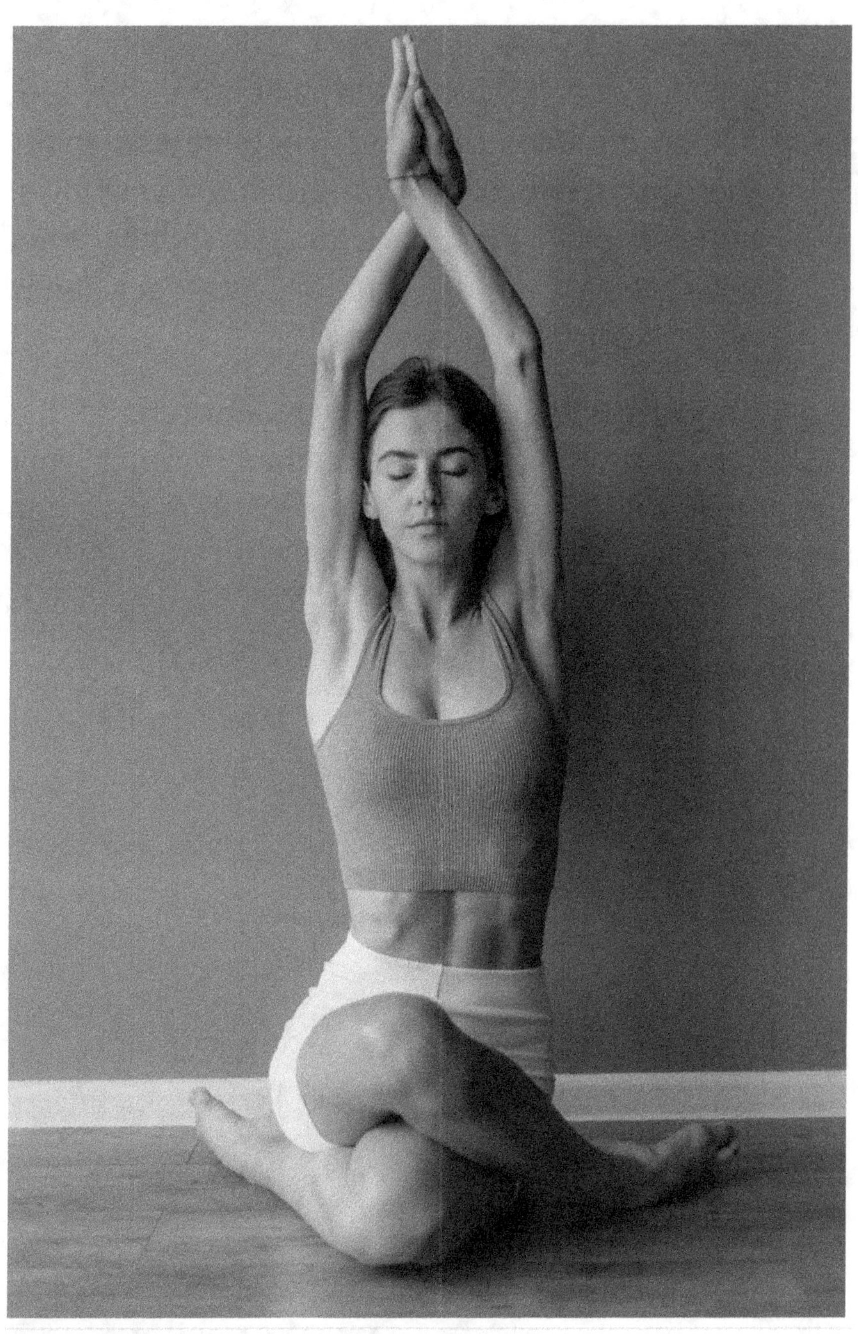

➢ **Seated Forward Fold with Side Stretch:** Sit towards the front of your chair with your feet flat on the floor. Inhale to lengthen your spine, then exhale to hinge forward from your hips, bringing your chest towards your thighs. Hold onto the sides of the chair or place your hands on your shins for support.

As you exhale, reach your right arm towards the left side of the room, stretching through your right side body. Hold for several breaths, then switch sides.

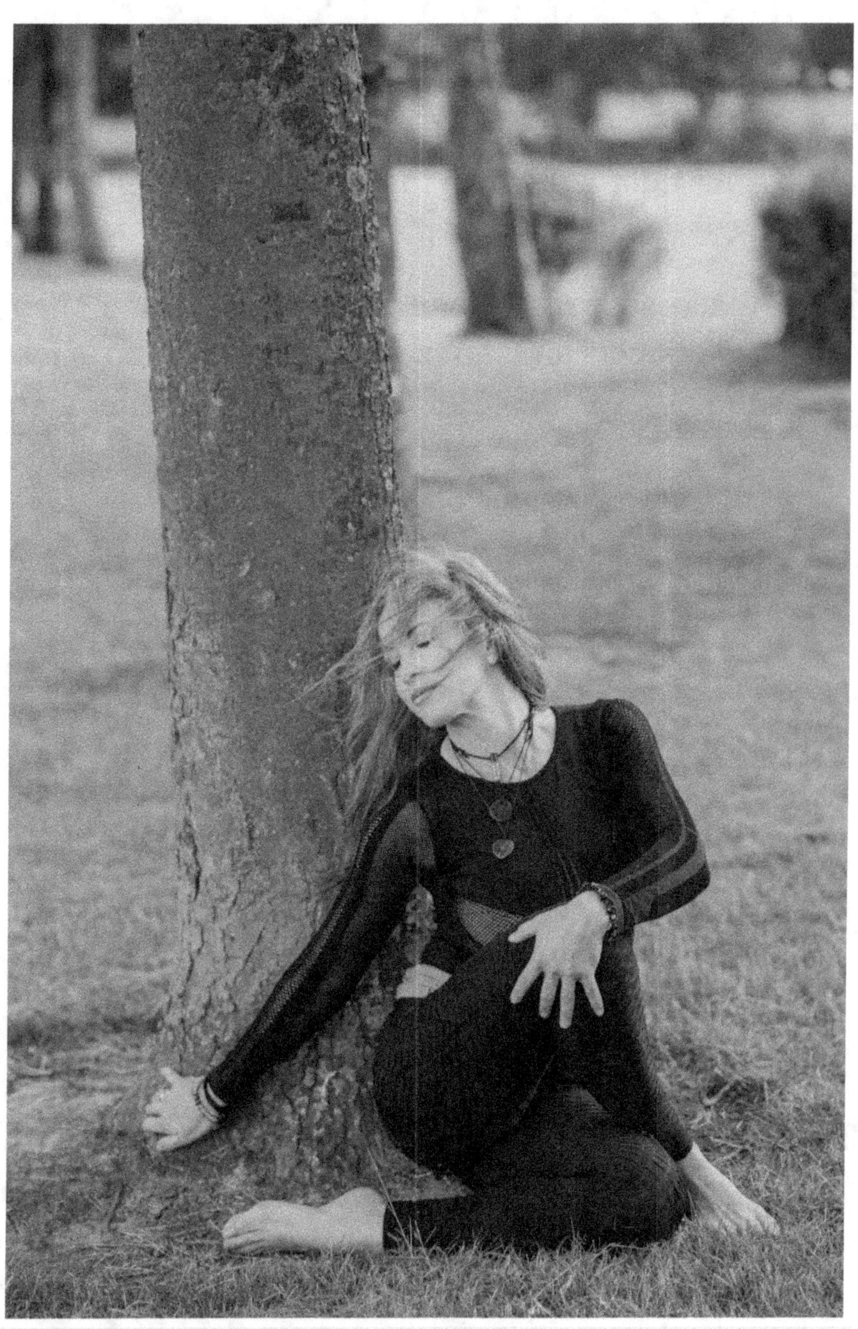

➢ **Seated Half Moon Pose:** Sit towards the front of your chair with your feet flat on the floor. Extend your right leg out to the side, keeping your foot flexed and your toes pointing forward.

Place your right hand on the seat of the chair for support and reach your left arm up towards the ceiling. Inhale to lengthen your spine, then exhale to side bend towards the right, creating a stretch through your left side body.

Hold for several breaths, then switch sides.

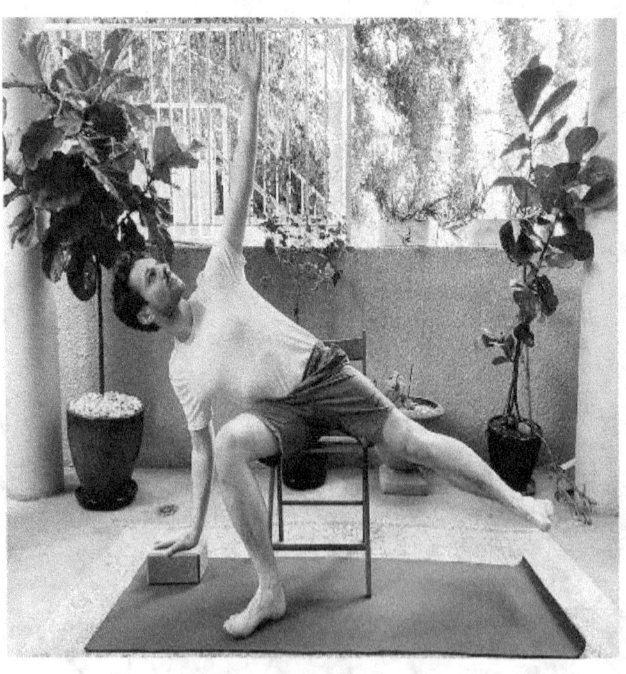

- ➢ **Seated Figure Four Pose:** Sit towards the front of your chair with your feet flat on the floor. Cross your right ankle over your left knee, flexing your right foot to protect your knee. Keep your spine tall and gently press your right knee towards the floor, feeling a stretch through your right hip and outer thigh. Hold for several breaths, then switch sides.

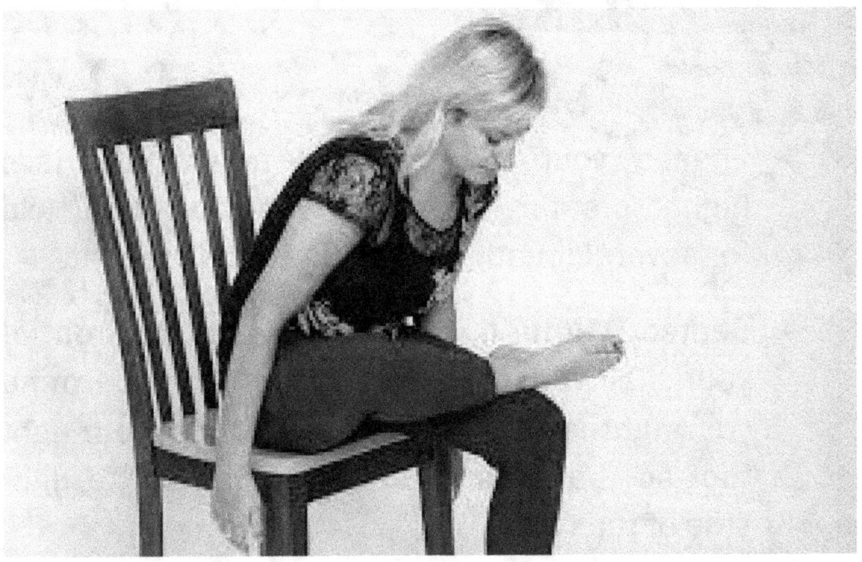

- ➢ **Seated Boat Pose:** Sit towards the front of your chair with your feet flat on the floor. Hold onto the sides of the chair for support and lean back slightly, lifting your feet off the floor.

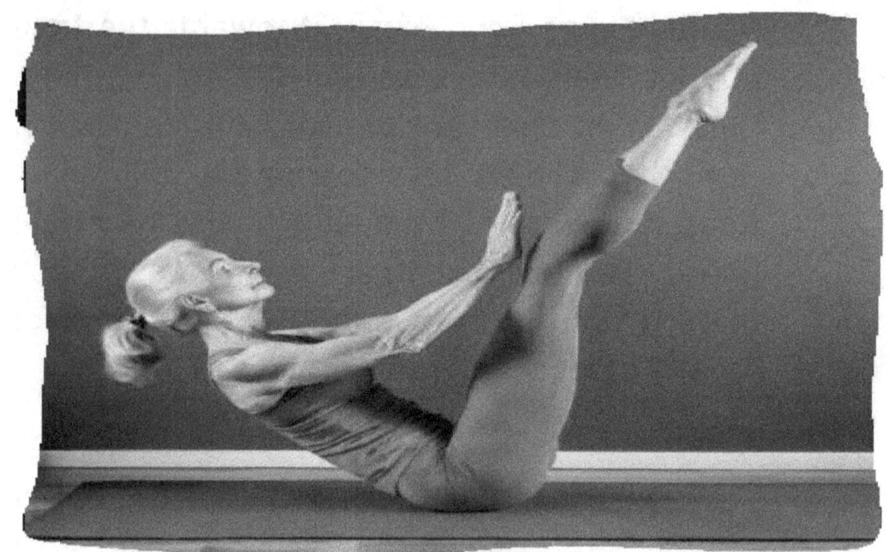

- ➤ Engage your core muscles to lift your legs higher, creating a V-shape with your body. Hold for several breaths, then release and repeat.

- ➤ Seated Warrior II Pose: Sit towards the front of your chair with your feet flat on the floor. Extend your right leg out to the side and turn your right foot so that your toes point towards the right side of the room.

- ➤ Keep your left foot grounded and your spine tall. Bend your right knee and bring your right forearm to rest on your right thigh, reaching your left arm up towards the ceiling. Gaze past your left fingertips and hold for several breaths, then switch sides.

As you explore these advanced chair yoga poses for seniors, remember to listen to your body and honor its limits. Pay attention to any sensations of discomfort or strain, and modify the poses as needed to suit your individual needs. With consistent practice and patience, you can continue to deepen your yoga practice and experience the many benefits it has to offer.

3.2 Ideal Chair Yoga Poses for Beginners

For seniors who are new to chair yoga, it's essential to start with gentle poses that promote flexibility, mobility, and relaxation. Ideal chair yoga positions for beginners offer a gentle introduction to the practice, helping seniors build confidence and ease into their yoga practice.

Here are some ideal chair yoga positions for beginners to try:

> ➤ Seated Mountain Pose: Sit tall in your chair with your feet flat on the floor and your spine straight. Place your hands on your thighs or knees, palms facing down. Close your eyes and take several deep breaths, grounding down through your sit bones and reaching up through

the crown of your head. This pose helps improve posture and awareness of alignment.

- ➢ **Seated Cat-Cow Pose:** Sit towards the front of your chair with your feet flat on the floor and your hands resting on your knees. Inhale to arch your back and lift your chest forward, opening your heart towards the ceiling (Cow Pose). Exhale to round your spine and tuck your chin towards your chest, drawing your navel towards your spine (Cat Pose). Repeat this flowing movement several times, moving with your breath.

- ➢ **Seated Forward Fold:** Sit towards the front of your chair with your feet flat on the floor and your spine tall. Inhale to lengthen your spine, then exhale to hinge forward from your hips, bringing your chest towards your thighs. Keep your back flat and your neck in line with your spine. Hold onto the sides of the chair or rest your hands on your shins for support. This pose helps stretch the spine, hamstrings, and lower back.

- ➢ **Seated Twist:** Sit towards the front of your chair with your feet flat on the floor and your spine tall. Place your right hand on the outside of your left knee and your left hand on the back of the chair. Inhale to lengthen your spine, then exhale to twist towards the left, gazing over your left shoulder. Hold for several breaths, then switch sides. This pose helps improve spinal mobility and digestion.

- ➢ **Seated Side Bend:** Sit towards the front of your chair with your feet flat on the floor and your spine tall. Inhale to lengthen your spine, then exhale to lean towards the right, bringing your right hand down towards the floor and reaching your left arm up and over your head. Hold for several breaths, then switch sides. This pose helps stretch the side body and improve lateral mobility.

- ➢ **Seated Butterfly Pose:** Sit towards the front of your chair with your feet flat on the floor and your knees bent. Bring the soles of your feet together and let your knees fall open to the sides, forming a diamond shape with your legs. Hold onto your ankles or shins, and gently press your knees towards the floor. This pose helps open the hips and inner thighs, promoting relaxation and flexibility.

➢ Seated Ankle Rolls: Sit towards the front of your chair with your feet flat on the floor. Lift one foot off the floor and begin to rotate your ankle in circles, moving in one direction and then the other. Continue for several rotations, then switch to the other foot. This pose helps improve ankle mobility and circulation in the feet and lower legs.

➢ Seated Shoulder Rolls: Sit towards the front of your chair with your feet flat on the floor and your hands resting on your knees. Inhale to lift your shoulders up towards your ears, then exhale to roll them back and down. Continue for several rotations, then switch directions. This pose helps release tension in the shoulders and neck, promoting relaxation and stress relief.

As you explore these ideal chair yoga positions for beginners, remember to move with awareness and breath, listening to your body's signals and modifying poses as needed to suit your individual needs. With consistent practice and patience, you can gradually build strength, flexibility, and balance, enjoying the many benefits of chair yoga for seniors.

3.3 Chair Yoga for Intermediate Level

For seniors who have been practicing chair yoga for a while and are ready to explore more challenging poses and sequences, intermediate-level chair yoga offers an opportunity to deepen your practice and continue to grow. Chair yoga for intermediate level introduces more advanced poses and sequences that build strength, flexibility, and balance, while also promoting mindfulness and relaxation.

Here are some chair yoga poses and sequences for intermediate-level practitioners to try:

- **Seated Warrior I Pose**: Sit towards the front of your chair with your feet flat on the floor and your spine tall. Extend your right leg back behind you and place the ball of your right foot on the floor, toes pointing forward.

- Keep your left knee bent and your left foot flat on the floor. Inhale to reach your arms overhead, palms facing each other.

- Exhale to sink deeper into your left knee, feeling a stretch through the front of your right hip and thigh. Hold for several breaths, then switch sides.

> **Seated Warrior II Pose:** Sit towards the front of your chair with your feet flat on the floor and your spine tall. Extend your right leg out to the side and turn your right foot so that your toes point towards the right side of the room.

> **WATCH VIDEO FOR THE WARRIOR POSES:** https://www.youtube.com/watch?v=flxNw-xXeME

> Keep your left foot grounded and your spine tall. Bend your right knee and bring your right forearm to rest on your right thigh, reaching your left arm up towards the ceiling.

> Gaze past your left fingertips and hold for several breaths, then switch sides. This pose strengthens the legs, improves balance, and promotes concentration.

> **Seated Tree Pose:** Sit towards the front of your chair with your feet flat on the floor and your spine tall. Lift your right foot off the floor and place the sole of your right foot against your left inner thigh or calf, avoiding the knee.

➤ Press your right foot into your leg and your leg into your foot, finding balance and stability. Bring your hands to your heart center or reach them overhead. Hold for several breaths, then switch sides. This pose improves balance, concentration, and stability.

➤ **Seated Extended Side Angle Pose:** Sit towards the front of your chair with your feet flat on the floor and your spine tall. Extend your right leg out to the side and turn your right foot so that your toes point towards the right side of the room. Keep your left foot grounded and your spine tall. Bend your right knee and bring your right forearm to rest on your right thigh, reaching your left arm up and over your head. Gaze towards your left fingertips and hold for several breaths, then switch sides. This pose stretches the side body, strengthens the legs, and improves flexibility.

➤ **Seated Boat Pose Variation:** Sit towards the front of your chair with your feet flat on the floor and your spine tall. Hold onto the sides of the chair for support and lean back slightly, lifting your feet off the floor.

- Extend your arms out in front of you at shoulder height, palms facing each other. Engage your core muscles to lift your legs higher, creating a V-shape with your body.

- Hold for several breaths, then release. This pose strengthens the core, improves balance, and promotes stability.

- **Seated Camel Pose:** Sit towards the front of your chair with your feet flat on the floor and your spine tall. Place your hands on the back of the chair, fingers pointing downwards.

- Inhale to lift your chest and arch your back, opening your heart towards the ceiling.

- Keep your neck long and gaze towards the sky. Hold for several breaths, then release. This pose stretches the front of the body, opens the chest, and promotes emotional release.

- **Seated Garland Pose:** Sit towards the front of your chair with your feet flat on the floor and your spine tall. Bring your feet together and let your knees fall open to the sides, forming a diamond shape with your legs.

➢ Hold onto your ankles or shins, and gently press your knees towards the floor. Bring your hands to your heart center and lift your chest.

➢ Hold for several breaths, then release. This pose stretches the inner thighs, groin, and hips, and promotes relaxation.

➢ **Seated Warrior III Pose:** Sit towards the front of your chair with your feet flat on the floor and your spine tall.

➢ Extend your right leg out in front of you, keeping it parallel to the floor. Flex your right foot and engage your thigh muscles.

➢ Lean forward slightly, bringing your torso parallel to the floor, and extend your arms out in front of you at shoulder height, palms facing each other.

➢ Hold for several breaths, then switch sides. This pose strengthens the legs, improves balance, and promotes focus and concentration.

As you explore these intermediate-level chair yoga poses and sequences, remember to listen to your body and honor its limits. Pay attention to any sensations of discomfort or strain, and modify the poses as needed to suit your individual needs. With consistent practice and patience, you can continue to deepen your yoga practice and experience the many benefits it has to offer.

Chapter 4:

Embracing Breath Awareness

As you deepen your practice of chair yoga, it's essential to cultivate a strong connection to your breath.

Breath awareness is the foundation of yoga, serving as a powerful tool for calming the mind, reducing stress, and enhancing your overall well-being.

Begin by sitting comfortably in your chair, eyes closed and hands resting on your lap.

Take a moment to simply observe your breath, noticing its natural rhythm and flow.

Pay attention to the sensation of the breath as it enters and leaves your body, the rise and fall of your chest, and the subtle movements that accompany each inhale and exhale.

Now, bring your awareness to the quality of your breath. Is it shallow or deep? Smooth or jagged? Without trying to change anything, simply observe the breath as it is in this moment. As you continue to breathe, gradually begin to deepen your inhales and exhales, allowing the breath to become slow, steady, and smooth.

With each inhale, imagine drawing in fresh energy and vitality, filling your body with light and positivity. With each exhale, imagine releasing any tension, stress, or negativity, allowing it to dissolve into the space around you.

Use your breath as a tool for letting go of anything that no longer serves you, creating space for peace and relaxation to enter. As you deepen your breath awareness, you may notice a sense of calmness and clarity washing over you.

Allow yourself to surrender to the present moment, letting go of any worries or distractions. With each breath, come home to yourself, finding refuge in the stillness and silence within.

In the next chapter, we'll explore specific breathing techniques that you can incorporate into your chair yoga practice to enhance relaxation, reduce anxiety, and promote a greater sense of well-being. Until then, continue to cultivate awareness of your breath, knowing that it is always there to guide you back to the present moment.

- **Myths about chair Yoga**

4.1 Perceived Chair Yoga Myths Vs Reality

Despite its growing popularity and proven benefits, chair yoga is sometimes subject to various myths and misconceptions. Let's debunk some of the common myths about chair yoga:

Myth 1: Chair yoga is only for seniors or people with limited mobility.

Reality: While chair yoga is indeed accessible and beneficial for seniors and individuals with limited mobility, it is suitable for people of all ages and abilities.

Chair yoga can be adapted to meet the needs of diverse populations, including those recovering from injuries, pregnant individuals, office workers, and anyone looking for a gentle and accessible form of yoga.

Myth 2: Chair yoga is not as effective as traditional yoga.

Reality: Chair yoga offers many of the same benefits as traditional yoga, including improved flexibility, strength, balance, and relaxation. The use of a chair as a prop can provide added stability and support, making yoga more accessible to individuals who may find traditional yoga challenging. Chair yoga also incorporates breath-work and mindfulness practices, promoting overall well-being and stress reduction.

Myth 3: Chair yoga is too easy and not challenging enough.

Reality: While chair yoga may appear gentler compared to traditional yoga styles, it can be as challenging as you make it.

By exploring different poses, variations, and sequences, you can customize your chair yoga practice to suit your needs and level of fitness. Chair yoga can also be adapted to target specific areas of the body or address individual health concerns, making it both accessible and versatile.

Myth 4: Chair yoga is only for relaxation and cannot provide a workout.

Reality: Chair yoga can be as dynamic or restorative as you choose to make it. By incorporating flowing sequences, strength-building poses, and breath-centered movements, you can create a chair yoga practice that offers a full-body workout.

Chair yoga can help improve muscle tone, cardiovascular health, and range of motion, making it a valuable addition to any fitness routine.

Myth 5: You need special equipment to practice chair yoga.

Reality: While props such as chairs, blocks, and straps can enhance your chair yoga practice, they are not essential. Many chair yoga poses can be done with just a sturdy chair and a clear space to move.

Chairs with armrests and stable bases are ideal for support and stability, but any sturdy chair will suffice. As you become more familiar with chair yoga, you can experiment with different props to enhance your practice.

By dispelling these common myths about chair yoga, we can recognize its value as a versatile and accessible form of yoga that offers numerous benefits for physical, mental, and emotional well-being.

4.2 The Feet and Toes Exercises Using Chair Yoga

The feet and toes are often overlooked in fitness routines, but they play a crucial role in balance, mobility, and overall health. Chair yoga offers a variety of exercises to strengthen and stretch the feet and toes, promoting better posture, stability, and foot health.

Here are some chair yoga exercises for the feet and toes:

- Toe Spread: Sit comfortably in your chair with your feet flat on the floor. Lift your toes off the ground and spread them apart as wide as you can. Hold for a few seconds, then release. Repeat several times, alternating between spreading your toes wide and relaxing them.

- Toe Flexion and Extension: Sit tall in your chair with your feet flat on the floor. Inhale as you flex your toes towards the ceiling, pointing them upwards as much as possible.

- Exhale as you curl your toes downwards, flexing them towards the floor. Repeat this movement several times, moving with your breath.

- Toe Tapping: Sit tall in your chair with your feet flat on the floor. Lift your toes off the ground and tap them lightly on the floor, one at a time, starting with your big toe and working towards your pinky toe. Continue tapping your toes for several rounds, then reverse the movement, tapping your toes from pinky to big toe.

- Heel Raises: Sit comfortably in your chair with your feet flat on the floor. Inhale as you lift your heels off the ground, rising up onto the balls of your feet. Exhale as you lower your heels back down to the floor. Repeat this movement several times, moving with your breath.

- Ankle Circles: Sit tall in your chair with your feet flat on the floor. Lift one foot off the ground and begin to circle your ankle in one direction, moving your foot through a full range of motion. After several circles, reverse the direction of the movement. Repeat on the other foot.

- Foot Stretch: Sit tall in your chair with your feet flat on the floor. Place a small ball or rolled-up towel under one foot. Roll the ball or towel back and forth under your foot, massaging the arch and heel. Switch to the other foot and repeat.

- Toe Stretch: Sit tall in your chair with your feet flat on the floor. Cross one ankle over the opposite knee, flexing the foot to protect the knee. Gently press down on the toes of the crossed foot, stretching the top of the foot and toes. Hold for a few breaths, then switch to the other foot.

- Sole Stretch: Sit tall in your chair with your feet flat on the floor. Lift one foot off the ground and place the sole of the foot on the opposite thigh. Hold onto your toes with one hand and gently press down on the toes with the other hand, stretching the sole of the foot. Hold for a few breaths, then switch to the other foot.

By incorporating these chair yoga exercises for the feet and toes into your daily routine, you can improve foot mobility, strength, and flexibility, leading to better balance, posture, and overall foot health.

4.3 Neck Circles

Neck circles are a simple and effective way to release tension in the neck and shoulders, improve mobility, and promote relaxation.

Chair yoga offers a modified version of neck circles that can be done comfortably while seated, making it accessible to individuals of all ages and abilities.

Here's how to practice neck circles in a chair:

- Sit comfortably in your chair with your feet flat on the floor and your spine tall.

- Take a few deep breaths to center yourself and relax your body.

- Gently drop your chin towards your chest, lengthening the back of your neck.

- Slowly begin to circle your head to the right, bringing your right ear towards your right shoulder, then gently rolling your head back, bringing your chin towards the ceiling, and finally bringing your left ear towards your left shoulder.

- Continue circling your head in this direction several times, moving with your breath and focusing on releasing tension in the neck and shoulders.

- After several circles, reverse the direction of the movement, circling your head to the left.

- Continue circling your head in this direction several times, moving with your breath and allowing any tension or tightness to melt away.

- After several circles, return your head to a neutral position and take a few deep breaths, noticing any sensations in your neck and shoulders.

By practicing neck circles regularly, you can improve neck mobility, reduce stiffness and discomfort, and promote relaxation and stress relief.

Remember to move slowly and mindfully, listening to your body and honoring its limits. If you experience any pain or discomfort during the practice, gently come out of the pose and adjust as needed.

4.4 Benefits of Neck Circles

Neck circles offer a range of benefits for both physical and mental well-being.

Here are some of the key benefits of practicing neck circles:

- Relieves Tension: Neck circles help to release tension and tightness in the neck and shoulders, which can build up due to poor posture, stress, or prolonged periods of sitting or standing.

- Improves Mobility: By gently moving the head through a circular motion, neck circles help to improve the range of motion in the neck joints, promoting flexibility and mobility.

- **Reduces Stiffness:** Regular practice of neck circles can help to alleviate stiffness in the neck and shoulders, making it easier to move the head and neck without discomfort.

- **Promotes Relaxation:** The gentle, rhythmic movement of neck circles can induce a sense of relaxation and calm, helping to reduce stress and anxiety.

- **Enhances Circulation:** Neck circles stimulate blood flow to the neck and shoulder muscles, which can help to alleviate tension and promote healing.

- **Improves Posture:** By releasing tension and tightness in the neck and shoulders, neck circles can help to improve overall posture, reducing the likelihood of developing forward head posture or rounded shoulders.

- **Relieves Headaches:** Neck circles can help to relieve tension headaches by releasing tight muscles in the neck and shoulders that may contribute to headache pain.

➢ **Promotes Mindfulness:** Practicing neck circles mindfully, focusing on the sensations in the body and the movement of the breath, can help to cultivate present-moment awareness and mindfulness.

Overall, neck circles are a simple yet effective way to promote neck and shoulder health, improve mobility and flexibility, and enhance overall well-being. By incorporating neck circles into your daily routine, you can experience these benefits and enjoy greater comfort and ease in your body and mind.

4.5 Shoulder Stretch

Shoulder stretches are essential for maintaining flexibility, mobility, and overall shoulder health. Chair yoga offers a variety of shoulder stretches that can be done comfortably while seated, making them accessible to individuals of all ages and abilities.

Here are some chair yoga shoulder stretches to try:

➢ **Shoulder Rolls:** Sit comfortably in your chair with your feet flat on the floor and your spine tall. Inhale as you lift your shoulders up towards your ears, then exhale as you roll them back and down. Repeat this movement several times, moving with your breath and focusing on releasing tension in the shoulders.

➢ Eagle Arms: Sit tall in your chair and reach your arms out to the sides at shoulder height. Cross your right arm over your left, bringing the backs of your hands together or wrapping your arms around each other until your palms touch. Lift your elbows slightly and feel a stretch across your upper back and shoulders. Hold for several breaths, then switch sides.

➢ Shoulder Stretch: Sit towards the front of your chair with your feet flat on the floor. Reach your right arm across your chest and place your hand on your left shoulder.

➢ Use your left hand to gently press your right elbow towards your chest, feeling a stretch in the back of your right shoulder.

➢ Hold for several breaths, then switch sides.

➢ Cow Face Arms: Sit tall in your chair and extend your right arm up towards the ceiling. Bend your right elbow and reach your right hand down your upper back, palm facing away from your body. Reach your left arm behind your back and bend your left elbow, bringing your left hand up towards your right hand.

➢ If possible, clasp your hands together or use a strap to connect them. Hold for several breaths, then switch sides.

➢ Reverse Prayer Pose: Sit tall in your chair and bring your hands behind your back, palms together in a prayer position. If possible, press your palms together and lift them up towards the ceiling, feeling a stretch across the front of your shoulders and chest. Hold for several breaths, then release.

➢ Thread the Needle: Sit towards the front of your chair with your feet flat on the floor. Reach your right arm underneath your left arm and thread it through the space between your left arm and torso, placing your right shoulder and ear on the floor.

➢ Press your left hand into the floor to deepen the stretch in your right shoulder. Hold for several breaths, then switch sides.

- ➢ Shoulder Opener: Sit tall in your chair and clasp your hands behind your back, interlacing your fingers. Inhale as you lift your chest and press your knuckles down towards the floor, opening your shoulders and chest. Hold for several breaths, then release.

- ➢ Supported Side Bend: Sit tall in your chair and extend your right arm up towards the ceiling. Place your left hand on the side of your chair and inhale as you lengthen your spine.

- ➢ Exhale as you lean to the left, stretching your right side body. Hold for several breaths, then switch sides.

By incorporating these chair yoga shoulder stretches into your daily routine, you can improve shoulder mobility, reduce tension and stiffness, and promote overall shoulder health.

Remember to move slowly and gently, listening to your body and honoring its limits. If you experience any pain or discomfort during the stretches, ease out of the pose and adjust as needed.

With consistent practice, you can enjoy greater comfort, flexibility, and ease of movement in your shoulder

Chapter 5

65 simple chair yoga poses for seniors over 70:

- Seated Mountain Pose: Sit up tall with your feet flat on the ground. Place your hands on your thighs and take deep breaths.

- Seated Forward Bend: Lean forward from your hips, reaching your hands towards your toes. Hold for a few breaths.

- Seated Cat-Cow Stretch: Place your hands on your knees. Inhale, arch your back, and look up. Exhale, round your spine, and look down.

- Seated Side Stretch: Raise your right arm and lean to the left. Hold and breathe. Repeat on the other side.

- Seated Twist: Place your left hand on the outside of your right thigh and twist to the right. Hold and breathe. Repeat on the other side.

- Seated Arm Circles: Extend your arms out to the sides and make small circles. Reverse direction after a few breaths.

- Seated Shoulder Shrugs: Lift your shoulders up towards your ears and then release them down.

- Seated Neck Stretch: Tilt your head to the right, bringing your ear towards your shoulder. Hold and breathe. Repeat on the other side.

- Seated Knee Lift: Lift one knee towards your chest, hold it with your hands, and breathe. Lower it and repeat with the other knee.

- Seated Ankle Rolls: Lift one foot and rotate your ankle in circles. Switch directions. Repeat with the other foot.

- Seated Leg Extension: Extend one leg out straight and hold. Lower it and repeat with the other leg.

Seated Toe Taps: Tap your toes on the floor and then lift them up. Repeat a few times.

Seated Heel Raises: Lift your heels off the floor and then lower them back down. Repeat a few times.

Seated Wrist Rolls: Extend your arms and rotate your wrists in circles. Switch directions.

Seated Finger Stretch: Spread your fingers wide apart and then close them into a fist. Repeat a few times.

- Seated Backbend: Place your hands on the back of your chair and gently arch your back, looking up towards the ceiling.

- Seated Shoulder Stretch: Bring your right arm across your chest and hold it with your left hand. Switch sides.

- Seated Chest Opener: Clasp your hands behind your back and lift them slightly as you open your chest.

- Seated Hamstring Stretch: Extend one leg out straight and reach for your toes. Hold and breathe. Switch legs.

- Seated Thigh Squeeze: Squeeze a small pillow or yoga block between your knees and release. Repeat a few times.

- Seated Hip Opener: Cross one ankle over the opposite knee and gently press down on the crossed knee.

- Seated Foot Flex: Flex your foot up towards your face and then point your toes away. Repeat with the other foot.

- Seated Calf Stretch: Place your feet flat on the floor and press your heels down as you lift your toes up.

- Seated Eagle Arms: Wrap your right arm under your left and lift your elbows. Hold and switch sides.

- Seated Spinal Twist: Cross your right knee over your left and twist to the left. Hold and switch sides.

- Seated Chair Pose: Sit slightly forward on your chair, lift your arms up, and hold as if sitting in an imaginary chair.

- Seated Tree Pose: Place one foot on the inside of the opposite thigh or calf, hold your hands together in front of your chest.

- Seated Warrior I: Sit sideways on your chair, extend one leg back, and raise your arms overhead. Switch sides.

- Seated Warrior II: Sit sideways on your chair, extend one leg back, and extend your arms out to the sides. Switch sides.

- Seated Warrior III: Sit slightly forward, lift one leg back, and extend your arms forward. Hold and switch sides.

- Seated Triangle Pose: Sit sideways, extend one leg out, reach one arm down towards your foot, and the other up. Switch sides.

- Seated Seated Side Bend: Extend your right arm up and over to the left, holding the chair with your left hand. Switch sides.

- Seated Forward Fold: Inhale deeply, then exhale as you fold forward, letting your hands reach towards the floor.

- Seated Chair Pigeon: Place your right ankle over your left knee, lean slightly forward. Switch sides.

- Seated Arm Reach: Extend one arm up and reach towards the ceiling. Hold and switch sides.

- Seated Side Arm Lift: Raise both arms to the sides, parallel to the floor. Hold and breathe.

- Seated Shoulder Blade Squeeze: Pull your shoulder blades together and hold, then release.

- Seated Arm Stretch: Reach your right arm behind your head and touch the back of your neck. Use your left hand to gently press. Switch sides.

- Seated Chest Stretch: Place your hands on your lower back and gently push your chest forward.

- Seated Core Twist: Sit up tall and gently twist from your waist to one side. Hold and switch sides.

- Seated Half Moon Pose: Extend both arms overhead and lean to one side. Hold and switch sides.

- Seated Shoulder Rolls: Roll your shoulders forward a few times, then roll them backward.

- Seated Gentle Backbend: Lean back slightly, placing your hands on your thighs for support.

- Seated Pelvic Tilt: Gently rock your pelvis forward and back while sitting up tall.

- Seated Inner Thigh Stretch: Place your feet wider than hip-width and lean slightly forward, keeping your back straight.

- Seated Outer Thigh Stretch: Cross one leg over the other and gently press the crossed knee with your hand.

- Seated Heel Press: Press your heels into the floor and hold for a few breaths.

- Seated Toe Spread: Spread your toes wide apart and then bring them back together.

- Seated Ankle Flexion: Flex your ankles up and down, alternating between feet.

- Seated Gentle Hug: Wrap your arms around yourself and give a gentle hug.

- Seated Elbow Circles: Place your hands on your shoulders and make circles with your elbows.

- Seated Thigh Lifts: Lift one thigh up towards your chest, hold, and lower it. Repeat with the other thigh.

- Seated Shoulder Opener: Place your hands on your shoulders and gently push your elbows back.

- Seated Wrist Flexion: Extend your arms out and flex your wrists up and down.

- Seated Neck Rolls: Gently roll your head in a circle. Switch directions after a few rolls.

- Seated Belly Breathing: Place your hands on your belly and take deep breaths, feeling your belly rise and fall.

- Seated Hand Stretch: Extend one arm out, palm facing up, and gently pull back on your fingers with the other hand.

- Seated Chest Expansion: Interlace your fingers behind your back and lift your hands slightly.

- Seated Leg Lift: Lift one leg straight up in front of you, hold, and lower it. Repeat with the other leg.

- Seated Hip Circles: Make small circles with your hips while sitting on the chair.

- Seated Inner Thigh Squeeze: Squeeze a pillow or yoga block between your thighs.

- Seated Outer Hip Stretch: Place one ankle over the opposite knee and gently press down on the raised knee.

- Seated Shoulder Flexion: Extend your arms straight out in front of you and raise them up towards the ceiling.

- Seated Shoulder Extension: Extend your arms straight out behind you and lift them slightly.

- **Seated Gentle Stretch:** Sit back in your chair, close your eyes, and take a few deep breaths, relaxing your body.

Enjoy your chair yoga practice!

Chapter 6:

Cultivating Relaxation and Meditation

AS you deepen your practice of chair yoga, it's essential to incorporate relaxation and meditation techniques to calm the mind, reduce stress, and promote a greater sense of well-being.

In this chapter, we'll explore how to cultivate relaxation and meditation in a seated position, allowing you to find peace and tranquility amidst the busyness of life.

Begin by finding a comfortable seated position in your chair, feet flat on the ground, and hands resting on your thighs. Close your eyes and take a few deep breaths, allowing your body to relax and soften with each exhale. As you continue to breathe, bring your awareness to the present moment, letting go of any worries or distractions.

Now, let's explore a simple relaxation technique known as progressive muscle relaxation. Begin by tensing the muscles in your feet and lower legs as tightly as you can, holding for a few seconds, and then releasing completely. Notice the sensation of relaxation spreading through your body as you let go of tension in each muscle group. Continue this process, working your way up through your body – calves, thighs, hips, abdomen, chest, arms, shoulders, neck, and face – until you've relaxed every muscle from head to toe.

Next, let's explore a seated meditation practice to quiet the mind and cultivate inner peace. Close your eyes and bring your awareness to your breath, allowing it to become slow, steady, and rhythmic.

As thoughts arise, simply acknowledge them without judgment and gently return your focus to the sensation of your breath. With each inhale, imagine drawing in light and positivity, and with each exhale, imagine releasing any tension or stress that no longer serves you.

Allow yourself to sink deeper into a state of relaxation with each breath, surrendering to the present moment with an open heart and mind.

Continue to explore relaxation and meditation practices in your chair yoga practice, knowing that these techniques are powerful tools for nurturing your body, mind, and spirit. With dedication and practice, you'll cultivate a greater sense of peace, clarity, and well-being in your daily life.

Chapter 7:
Taking Your Practice off the Chair

Here, we'll explore how to take the principles and benefits of chair yoga off the chair and into your everyday life.

While your chair yoga practice offers a sanctuary for self-care and reflection, it's equally important to integrate mindfulness and movement into your daily routine.

Begin by bringing awareness to your posture and alignment throughout the day. Whether you're sitting at your desk, standing in line at the grocery store, or walking through your neighborhood, pay attention to how you hold your body.

Aim to maintain a tall spine, relaxed shoulders, and engaged core muscles, supporting your body in optimal alignment.

As you go about your daily activities, take moments to pause and check in with your breath. Notice if it's shallow or deep, fast or slow.

If you notice any signs of tension or stress, take a few deep breaths to center yourself and create a sense of calmness and presence.

Incorporate gentle movement breaks into your day to release tension and rejuvenate your body. Whether it's stretching your arms overhead, rolling your shoulders back, or taking a short walk around your home or office, find opportunities to move mindfully and with intention.

Practice mindfulness in everyday tasks, such as eating, washing dishes, or walking. Bring your full attention to the present moment, savoring the sights, sounds, and sensations around you.

Notice the taste and texture of your food, the warmth of the water on your hands, or the feeling of the ground beneath your feet.

Find moments of stillness and quiet amidst the hustle and bustle of daily life. Whether it's taking a few minutes to sit in silence before starting your day or enjoying a peaceful cup of tea in the evening, carve out time for reflection and introspection.

As you continue to integrate the principles of chair yoga into your daily life, you'll find that mindfulness, movement, and breath awareness become second nature. These practices offer a pathway to greater balance, presence, and well-being, enriching every moment of your journey.

Embracing the Spirit of Community

While your practice may often be a solitary endeavor, there's great value in connecting with others who share your passion for health, wellness, and self-care.

Consider joining a local chair yoga class or community group where you can practice with others in a supportive and welcoming environment. These classes offer an opportunity to learn from experienced instructors, connect with like-minded individuals, and share in the joys and challenges of your yoga journey.

If attending in-person classes isn't feasible, explore virtual options such as online classes, forums, or social media groups dedicated to chair yoga. These virtual communities provide a platform for sharing resources, asking questions, and connecting with fellow practitioners from around the world.

In addition to formal classes and groups, consider reaching out to friends, family members, or neighbors who may be interested in exploring chair yoga with you. Organize informal gatherings or practice sessions where you can come together to support and uplift one another on your journey to health and wellness.

Remember that the spirit of community extends beyond the walls of a yoga studio or virtual space. Look for opportunities to give back to your community through acts of service, volunteer work, or supporting local charities and organizations. By contributing to the well-being of others, you'll deepen your sense of connection and fulfillment.

As you embrace the spirit of community in your chair yoga journey, you'll find that you're not alone on the path to health and wellness. Together, we can uplift and inspire one another, creating a ripple effect of positivity and compassion that extends far beyond the confines of our individual practices.

Chapter 8:

Nurturing Self-Compassion and Gratitude

ere we will also explore the transformative power of self-compassion and gratitude in your chair yoga practice.

As you navigate the ups and downs of life, cultivating a kind and loving relationship with yourself is essential for fostering resilience, inner peace, and well-being.

Begin by bringing awareness to your inner dialogue and how you speak to yourself. Notice if your thoughts are filled with self-criticism, judgment, or negativity. Whenever you catch yourself engaging in negative self-talk, gently redirect your thoughts with kindness and compassion. Offer yourself words of encouragement, love, and support, just as you would to a dear friend or loved one.

Practice gratitude as a daily ritual, taking time each day to reflect on the blessings and abundance in your life. Keep a gratitude journal where you can write down three things you're thankful for each day, no matter how big or small. Cultivate an attitude of appreciation for the simple joys, moments of beauty, and acts of kindness that grace your life each day.

Incorporate self-care practices into your daily routine, nourishing your body, mind, and soul with activities that bring you joy and fulfillment.

Whether it's taking a warm bath, spending time in nature, or indulging in a favorite hobby, prioritize activities that replenish your energy and uplift your spirit.

Practice forgiveness and letting go of past hurts or resentments, both towards yourself and others. Holding onto anger or resentment only weighs you down and prevents you from fully embracing the present moment.

Choose to release the burden of the past and cultivate a sense of freedom and liberation in the here and now.

As you nurture self-compassion and gratitude in your chair yoga practice, you'll discover a profound sense of acceptance, peace, and wholeness within yourself. Remember that you are worthy of love and compassion exactly as you are, and that your journey to health and wellness is a sacred and beautiful unfolding

Embracing Your Journey

ith all said and done, celebrate the culmination of your chair yoga journey and reflect on the growth, Wtransformation, and empowerment you've experienced along the way.

As you look back on your journey, take a moment to honor yourself for showing up, committing to your practice, and embracing the gift of self-care and self-discovery.

Acknowledge the progress you've made, both physically and emotionally, since embarking on your chair yoga journey. Notice how your body feels stronger, more flexible, and more vibrant with each passing day.

Recognize the shifts in your mindset and perspective, as you cultivate greater awareness, acceptance, and gratitude for yourself and others.

Celebrate the moments of courage and resilience that have carried you through challenges and obstacles on your path. Whether it's overcoming physical limitations, navigating life transitions, or facing inner fears and doubts, honor the strength and courage that resides within you.

Express gratitude for the teachers, mentors, and fellow practitioners who have supported and inspired you along the way.

From experienced instructors who've shared their wisdom and guidance to fellow practitioners who've offered encouragement and camaraderie, cherish the connections and community that have enriched your chair yoga journey.

As you embrace the fullness of your journey, take a moment to set intentions for the road ahead. What do you envision for yourself moving forward? How will you continue to nourish your body, mind, and spirit with the practices of chair yoga?

Trust in your inner wisdom and intuition, knowing that you have everything you need to create a life of health, happiness, and fulfillment.

21-Day Chair Yoga Fat Burn Challenge for Seniors Over 70

When it comes to burning fat and staying healthy as a senior, yoga can be your gentle yet effective ally. As you age, your metabolism naturally slows down, making it harder to maintain a healthy weight. But don't worry, because yoga offers you a powerful solution.

With its low-impact movements and customizable poses, yoga is accessible to you at any fitness level.

Chair yoga, especially, is tailored to meet your needs. It allows you to practice yoga comfortably while seated or using a chair for support. This form of yoga still delivers all the benefits of traditional yoga, like increased flexibility, toned muscles, and better circulation, while reducing the risk of injury.

Yoga doesn't just help you physically; it supports your mental and emotional well-being too. By incorporating deep breathing techniques and meditation, yoga helps you manage stress and emotional eating habits. As you cultivate mindfulness and inner peace, you'll find it easier to make healthier choices and maintain a balanced lifestyle.

Plus, yoga helps you build lean muscle mass, which is key to revving up your metabolism and burning fat. With targeted poses that engage your core, legs, arms, and back, you'll strengthen and tone your body over time. And as you build muscle, you'll naturally burn more calories, even when you're resting.

The beauty of yoga lies in its holistic approach to health and wellness. Instead of focusing on quick fixes or restrictive diets, yoga encourages you to listen to your body, honor your limits, and practice self-compassion. By fostering a positive relationship with food, exercise, and body image, you can achieve lasting results and enjoy a healthier, happier life.

So whether you're practicing chair yoga at home or joining a group class at a studio, know that yoga is your partner in this journey towards better health. With each breath and each pose, you're taking steps towards a stronger, leaner, and more vibrant you. Embrace the practice, trust in your body, and watch as yoga transforms your life for the better.

Welcome to your 21-day journey towards rejuvenation, vitality, and fat burn through chair yoga! As a professional yoga coach specializing in senior wellness, I'm thrilled to guide you through this transformative experience. Over the next three weeks, we'll delve into a series of chair yoga practices specifically designed to help you shed unwanted fat, boost metabolism, enhance flexibility, and promote overall well-being.

Day 1-7: Building Foundation and Awareness

Your journey begins with laying a strong foundation and cultivating mindfulness. Take a seat comfortably on your chair, ensuring your feet are firmly planted on the ground and your spine is tall. Close your eyes and take a few deep breaths, allowing yourself to arrive fully in the present moment. With each inhale, imagine filling your body with fresh energy, and with each exhale, release any tension or stress.

We'll start with gentle warm-up exercises to awaken your body and prepare it for the journey ahead. From seated twists to shoulder rolls and neck stretches, these movements will help increase circulation, loosen tight muscles, and improve mobility.

Next, we'll flow through a series of chair yoga poses targeting different muscle groups while maintaining a focus on breath awareness. From forward folds to gentle backbends and side stretches, each pose will be accessible and modified to suit your needs.

Throughout this first week, pay close attention to how your body feels in each posture. Notice any areas of tension or resistance and breathe into them gently, allowing for release and relaxation. Remember, yoga is not about pushing yourself to the limit but rather about listening to your body and honoring its needs.

Day 8-14: Igniting the Fat-Burning Fire

As we enter the second week of our challenge, it's time to turn up the heat and ignite the fat-burning fire within. We'll incorporate dynamic movements and flowing sequences to boost metabolism, increase calorie burn, and stimulate digestion.

Begin each session with a few rounds of Sun Salutations adapted for the chair. These energizing sequences will get your heart pumping and your blood flowing, setting the stage for a calorie-torching practice.

From there, we'll explore more challenging chair yoga poses that target multiple muscle groups simultaneously. Chair squats, chair lunges, and chair plank variations will strengthen your lower body, core, and upper body while revving up your metabolism.

Incorporate dynamic transitions between poses to keep the energy flowing and maintain a steady pace throughout your practice. Remember to stay connected to your breath, using it as a guide to move gracefully from one posture to the next.

Throughout this week, you may notice your body starting to feel stronger, leaner, and more energized.

Celebrate these small victories and continue to fuel your motivation as you progress through the challenge.

Day 15-21: Deepening the Practice and Cultivating Balance

As we enter the final week of our journey, it's time to deepen our practice and cultivate balance both physically and mentally. We'll focus on refining alignment, exploring variations of familiar poses, and incorporating mindfulness techniques to enhance our overall well-being.

Start each session with a brief meditation or breathing exercise to center yourself and cultivate a sense of inner peace. This will help you approach your practice with clarity, focus, and intention.

Explore more advanced chair yoga poses such as chair twists, chair balances, and chair inversions, taking your practice to new heights while challenging your strength, stability, and flexibility.

As you move through these poses, remember to maintain a sense of ease and effortlessness, finding the perfect balance between strength and surrender. If a pose feels too challenging, don't hesitate to modify or skip it altogether, honoring your body's limitations and respecting its boundaries.

Throughout this final week, reflect on how far you've come since the beginning of the challenge. Notice any changes in your body, mind, and spirit, and take pride in your progress and accomplishments.

Congratulations on completing your 21-day chair yoga fat burn challenge! You've dedicated yourself to your health and well-being, and the results speak for themselves. Not only have you shed unwanted fat and boosted your metabolism, but you've also cultivated strength, flexibility, and balance both on and off the mat.

As you continue your journey beyond this challenge, remember to stay committed to your practice, listen to your body, and approach each day with an open heart and mind.

Whether it's through chair yoga, meditation, or other forms of self-care, prioritize your health and well-being every step of the way.

Thank you for allowing me to be a part of your journey, and may you continue to shine bright and radiate vitality in all that you do. Namaste.

In conclusion

Remember that your chair yoga journey is not a destination, but a sacred and ongoing process of growth and evolution. Embrace each moment with an open heart and a curious mind, knowing that every breath, every movement, and every moment of stillness is an opportunity to awaken to the fullness of your being.

As you move forward on your journey, remember to stay connected to the wisdom and teachings of chair yoga. Let the principles of mindfulness, breath awareness, and self-compassion be your guiding lights, illuminating your path and supporting you through life's twists and turns.

Continue to explore and deepen your practice, whether it's by trying new poses, attending classes or workshops, or simply dedicating time each day to sit in stillness and presence. Trust in the process of your practice, knowing that each step you take brings you closer to your true self.

Be gentle with yourself along the way, honoring your body's needs and limitations with compassion and understanding. Listen to the whispers of your heart and the wisdom of your body, allowing them to guide you towards choices that nourish and uplift you.

And most importantly, celebrate the journey itself – the highs and lows, the breakthroughs and setbacks, the moments of joy and the lessons learned. Every step you take, every breath you breathe, is a testament to your courage, resilience, and commitment to your own well-being.

As you embrace the fullness of your chair yoga journey, may you continue to shine brightly as a beacon of inspiration and possibility for other's.

May your practice be a source of strength, peace, and joy, not only for yourself but for all beings every where.

With gratitude and love, we honor the beauty and power of your chair yoga journey, knowing that the light you cultivate within yourself has the power to illuminate the world around you.

ABOUT THE AUTHOR

Dr. Sheila Douglas is a highly respected figure in the field of holistic health and wellness. With a Ph.D. in Integrative Medicine and over two decades of experience, Dr. Douglas has dedicated her career to empowering individuals to achieve optimal health through natural and sustainable means.

Dr. Douglas is not only a seasoned practitioner but also a passionate advocate for holistic living. Her journey into the world of holistic health began early in her career when she witnessed firsthand the limitations of conventional medicine in addressing the root causes of chronic illness and disease. This experience inspired her to explore alternative healing modalities, including yoga, meditation, nutrition.

Throughout her career, Dr. Douglas has conducted extensive research and clinical work in the field of integrative medicine. Her groundbreaking studies on the effects of yoga and mindfulness on health outcomes have been published in numerous peer-reviewed journals and have earned her recognition from the medical community.

As a yoga instructor and wellness coach, Dr. Douglas brings a unique blend of expertise and compassion to her work. She believes in meeting her clients where they are and tailoring her approach to their individual needs and goals. Whether working with seniors, athletes, or individuals managing chronic conditions,

Dr. Douglas emphasizes the importance of holistic health and lifestyle interventions in achieving long-term wellness.

In addition to her clinical practice, Dr. Douglas is a sought-after speaker and educator, sharing her knowledge and insights at conferences, workshops, and retreats around the world. She is known for her engaging and informative teaching style, which blends scientific evidence with practical wisdom and personal anecdotes.

Dr. Sheila Douglas is also the author of several bestselling books on holistic health and wellness, including "Unveiling Paranoid Personality Disorder" A Holistic Approach to overcoming paranoia." Her writing is renowned for its clarity, depth, and accessibility, making complex health concepts easy to understand and apply in everyday life.

Above all, Dr. Douglas is committed to empowering individuals to take control of their health and well-being and live their best lives possible. Through her work, she seeks to inspire others to embrace a holistic approach to health, one that honors the interconnectedness of mind, body, and spirit.